Drugs of Natural Origin
Economic and Policy Aspects of Discovery, Development, and Marketing

Drugs of Natural Origin
Economic and Policy Aspects of Discovery, Development, and Marketing

Anthony Artuso, PhD

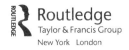

Routledge
Taylor & Francis Group
New York   London

First published by
The Haworth Press, Inc., 10 Alice Street, Binghamton, NY 13904-1580

This edition published 2012 by Routledge

Routledge
Taylor & Francis Group
711 Third Avenue
New York, NY 10017

Routledge
Taylor & Francis Group
2 Park Square, Milton Park
Abingdon, Oxon OX14 4RN

The development, preparation, and publication of this work has been undertaken with great care. However, the publisher, employees, editors, and agents of The Haworth Press are not responsible for any errors contained herein or for consequences that may ensue from use of materials or information contained in this work. The opinions expressed by the author(s) are not necessarily those of The Haworth Press, Inc.

Cover design by Monica L. Seifert.

Library of Congress Cataloging-in-Publication Data

Artuso, Anthony.
  Drugs of natural origin : economic and policy aspects of discovery, development, and marketing / Anthony Artuso.
       p.   cm.
  Includes bibliographical references and index.
  ISBN 0-7890-0123-3 (alk. paper). ISBN 0-7890-0414-3 (alk. paper).
  1. Pharmacognosy–Government policy. 2. Pharmacognosy–Economic aspects. 3. Biological diversity conservation–Economic aspects.   4. Biological diversity conservation–Government policy. 5. Pharmaceutical policy. I. Title.
RS169.A78   1997
615'.19–dc21
                                                                                97-19503
                                                                                CIP

CONTENTS

ABOUT THE AUTHOR

Anthony Artuso, PhD, is Assistant Professor of Public Policy at the University of Charleston, South Carolina. His current research interests include the value of biodiversity as a source of commercially valuable chemicals and genetic materials and international policy involved in implementation of the Convention on Biological Diversity. Dr. Artuso has served as an advisor to the National Institutes of Health, the Environmental Protection Agency, the Pan American Health Organization, and the World Bank. He is currently working with the United Nations Conference on Trade and Development on the BioTrade Initiative, a program designed to promote efficient and equitable international markets for biological resources.

Chapter 1

Biodiversity and the Search for New Drugs

INTRODUCTION

Access to novel biochemicals has become a valuable input in many research and development (R&D) processes. Individual genes, peptides, proteins, and other biochemical compounds have become an important source of innovation not only in the pharmaceutical industry but also in the development of agrochemicals, industrial feedstocks, cosmetics, fragrances, and flavors (Oldfield 1984; Klocke 1989; Myers 1992; Broad 1993). In the search for stronger, lighter, more durable materials, researchers have begun to unlock the secrets of spider silk, seashells, and reindeer antlers, and there are even indications that genetic material may provide the basis for a new wave of advances in computer technology (Leary 1993; Lipton 1995). Each of these activities can be considered an aspect of biochemical prospecting, which I shall refer to as the purposeful evaluation of biological material in search of economically valuable discoveries.

Perhaps the most well-publicized form of biochemical prospecting is the screening of biological extracts for novel chemical compounds that can provide leads in the development of new medicines. It is this area of research that is the principal focus of this book. However, I shall periodically remind the reader that the models, analytical techniques, and policy recommendations presented here are generally applicable to the broader spectrum of biochemical prospecting activities.

Only a small percentage of the world's plant and animal species have been systematically evaluated for their medicinal values.

Microorganisms, including bacteria and some classes of fungi, have received perhaps the most attention from pharmaceutical researchers, partly as a result of the impetus provided by the discovery of the antibiotic properties of the penicillium mold (Mitscher et al. 1987; Oldfield 1984, p. 122). Microorganisms have also been a favorite subject of pharmaceutical and biotechnological research because of the relative ease with which they can be manipulated and reproduced in the laboratory (Borris 1994). Yet even after several decades of intensive research, less than 5 percent of the estimated 5.4 million species of microorganisms have even been described, let alone evaluated for commercial value (Hawksworth 1992, pp. 47-48). Although higher plants have been relatively well-studied taxonomically, Farnsworth and Soejarto (1985) suggest that perhaps only 2 percent of the approximately 250,000 species of higher plants have been thoroughly evaluated as sources of new drugs. Insects, which comprise the majority of Earth's species, are perhaps the least well-inventoried group of organisms. Estimates of total species diversity range from 2 million to more than 50 million (May 1990; Stork 1988). The nearly one million scientifically described insect species have received relatively little attention as sources of new medicines (Grifo 1996, p. 7; Oldfield 1984, p. 126).

While nature has long been a source of new medicines and other valuable products, it is the more recent concern over the rate of species extinction that has caused biochemical prospecting to become a focus for politicians and policymakers. Interest in the potential connection between biochemical prospecting and biodiversity protection was heightened when Merck announced its contract with Costa Rica's Instituto Nacional de Biodiversidad (INBio) in 1991. The Merck-INBio contract attracted worldwide attention because it was perhaps the first to provide both advance compensation for biological samples and a share of the royalties generated from any new products derived from the venture. Merck also agreed to provide technical assistance and training, while INBio allocated a 10 percent share of the advance payments and 50 percent of any royalties to a fund established to support Costa Rica's National Park Service. The National Cancer Institute, Bristol-Myers Squibb, SmithKline Beecham, Glaxo, and Pfizer are a few other prospecting organizations that have also agreed to provide or negotiate royalties and other forms of compensation for access to biological material in countries such as China, Surinam, Peru, Argentina, Mexico, Chile, Nigeria, and Cameroon.

PROSPECTING LOCATIONS AND SPECIES EXTINCTION

From the perspective of biochemical prospecting, not all ecosystems are created equal. Humid tropical forests cover only 8 percent of the surface area of the continents but contain over 50 percent of all terrestrial species (FAO 1990; Harcourt 1992, p. 256). High temperatures, humidity, and species density, combined with a continuous growing season, have caused many rainforest species to develop complex chemical mechanisms for attraction of pollinators and mates and for defense against predators and parasites (Kricher 1989, pp. 180–210). These intra- and interspecies interactions can provide important leads in the search for valuable new chemical compounds. For example, numerous drugs and pesticides have been derived from alkaloids, phenols, saponins, and other secondary metabolites that serve as the chemical defenses of many tropical plant species (Oldfield 1984, pp. 95–110; Kricher 1989, pp. 180–192).

Unfortunately, over the past decade, humid tropical forests were being cleared at a rate of 170,000 square kilometers per year (Whitmore and Sayer 1992). Efforts to determine how tropical forest clearance is affecting the rate of species extinction have been hindered by poor information on the original number, taxonomic composition, and biogeographic distribution of tropical species. Most estimates of species extinction in the tropics are therefore based on the relationship between the size of an ecosystem and the number of species that are found within it (i.e., the species-area curve). Using various estimates of this relationship and a range of projections for future rates of deforestation in Asia, Africa, and Latin America, researchers have estimated that from 3 percent to perhaps as much as 15 percent of all species could become extinct within the next several decades (Reid 1992, p. 58).

Tropical humid forests are not the only ecosystems that offer productive sites for biochemical prospecting. Other ecosystems characterized by high species diversity, such as coral reefs, or by unique biological and physical stresses, such as deserts or deep ocean vents, are also the focus of ongoing biochemical prospecting activities. The National Cancer Institute (NCI) screens thousands of marine organisms each year, many of which are obtained from marine environments (National Cancer Institute 1994). Through the International Cooperative Biodiversity Group Program, the National Institutes of Health (NIH), in conjunction with the National Science Foundation and the U.S. Agency for International Development, are providing assistance for biochemical prospecting efforts in arid ecosystems in Chile, Argentina, and Mexico (Grifo 1996). The thermophilic organisms found in deep ocean vents and hot springs are being intensively explored by many biotechnology companies as a source of genetic material and other biochemicals that can be used in heat-intensive industrial and chemical processes (Broad 1993).

Even relatively well-explored or seemingly sterile ecosystems can yield important biochemical discoveries. Merck's ivermectin was developed from a compound produced by a fungi unearthed in the fairway of a golf course, and Merck is developing another broad-spectrum antibiotic from a microorganism found in the soil near the company's New Jersey headquarters (Caporale 1994). Nevertheless, with the possible exception of coral reefs, tropical rainforests may be subject to greater rates of habitat destruction and species extinction than any other major ecosystem type. In addition, countries in which the majority of the world's tropical forests are located generally have inadequate resources to devote to biodiversity.

ESTIMATING THE VALUE OF BIODIVERSITY FOR PHARMACEUTICAL R&D

The size of the market for biologically derived pharmaceutical products has raised hopes that biochemical prospecting, particularly natural product research by the pharmaceutical industry, could provide substantial economic incentives to protect biodiversity and provide biologically rich countries with an opportunity for sustainable development. A recent study found that, on the basis of the number of prescriptions filled each year, 57 percent of the top-selling 150 pharmaceutical products in 1993 contained active ingredients that were natural products, derivatives, or analogs of natural products (Grifo et al. 1996). Since sales of prescription drug products in 1990 were approximately $147 billion, biologically derived pharmaceuticals could reasonably generate in excess of $100 billion in revenues per year (USITC 1991). While this estimate provides some indication of the historical importance of biodiversity as a source of new drugs, it does not provide sufficient information on the value of preserving species for their pharmaceutical potential.

Despite growing international interest, there have been very few systematic efforts to estimate the value of biological resources as a source of new chemical compounds. Farnsworth and Soejarto (1985) were perhaps the first to estimate the cost of plant extinctions in terms of lost opportunities for new drug development. They estimate that extinction of flowering plants will result in forgone drug revenues in excess of $1.5 million per species per year in 1980 dollars. The critical assumption underlying this estimate is that one out of every 125 plants investigated will lead to a new drug discovery. Using a somewhat lower success rate (1/2,000), Principe (1989) extended Farnsworth and Soejarto's study to include foregone drug revenues in other developed countries. He concludes that each plant extinction will result in $300,000 of foregone new drug revenues. Unfortunately, the Farnsworth/Soejarto and Principe studies do not take into account the costs of new drug development or consider how alternatives to natural product research might affect their estimates of the foregone benefits resulting from plant extinctions. As a result, both studies tend to overestimate the value of preserving a species for pharmaceutical research.

Aylward (1993) and Mendelsohn and Balick (1995) have developed more useful estimates of the pharmaceutical value of rainforest species, which attempt to incorporate the cost of new drug development as well as potential revenues. Aylward estimates that the combined expected net present value to suppliers of biological samples and to the firm engaged in natural product research is approximately $4,000 per biological sample. Mendelsohn and Balick estimate the net present value of as yet undiscovered new drugs from rainforest plants to be approximately $147 billion, or $1.2 million per tropical plant species.[1] However, the net present value to any one pharmaceutical firm of obtaining exclusive rights to screen tropical plants is estimated to be less than $4.1 billion, or $32,800 per tropical plant species.

The divergence in the estimates of the value of biological samples generated by these two studies is due to two factors. First, Mendelsohn and Balick assume that one out of every one million plant samples tested in any given screening test will lead to a new drug and that each plant will yield six chemically distinct samples. In addition, they assume that there are over 500 statistically independent screening tests being employed by the pharmaceutical industry, although any single firm may have access to only 50 to 75 screens. Together, these assumptions imply that, on average, one new drug would be developed from every 333 rainforest plants that are thoroughly screened for pharmaceutical potential. Second, Aylward's analysis does not take into account the number of therapeutic targets for which each biological sample might be screened. He simply uses a success rate of one new drug per 10,000 samples tested and assumes that two distinct samples will be derived from each species, yielding a composite success rate of one new drug per 5,000 species tested. Mendelsohn and Balick also assume that for the industry as a whole, including makers of generic drugs, revenues from a new drug discovery rise steadily for the first ten years and then remain at this peak level indefinitely. Aylward's analysis includes only the revenues derived by the firm that patents the original discovery.

Neither Aylward nor Mendelsohn and Balick develop very detailed models of the pharmaceutical R&D process. In particular, both studies fail to consider the relationship between the cost of new drug development from biological material and the number of biological samples that must be tested to develop a new drug. In addition, Mendelsohn and Balick's assumption about the number of independent screens available to the pharmaceutical industry is particularly questionable. Since many of these proprietary screens are testing for activity in very similar therapeutic categories, the number of truly independent screens is likely to be greater than the 50 or so screens that they estimate any one firm employs but much lower than 500. This correction would proportionately reduce their estimate of the value of preserving any individual species. A countervailing consideration is that neither Mendelsohn and Balick nor Aylward attempts to include the full social benefits of new drug discovery or the option value of preserving a species for pharmaceutical research.

Simpson, Sedjo, and Reid (1996) make the very important point that these and other prior studies do not take into account the declining marginal value of biological samples to the pharmaceutical industry. In their model, the expected value of screening an additional sample declines due to the increasing probability of already having satisfied the demand for new drugs from samples already screened. They have attempted to show that if a pharmaceutical company were to obtain samples from all but 1 of the estimated 250,000 species of higher plants, the net present value of screening the remaining species of higher plants would be less than $9,500, even if the screening success rate is set to maximize the value of this marginal species.

Using a species-area curve model, Simpson and colleagues go on to demonstrate that with a value of $9,500 for the marginal species, the value of conserving natural habitat for purposes of pharmaceutical research—even in areas with the highest density of endemic plant species—is only $21 per hectare. Moreover, in their model, the value of the marginal species, and therefore the marginal hectare of natural ecosystems, declines rapidly if the actual success rate of natural product research differs from the level necessary to maximize the value of the marginal species. From this they conclude that biochemical prospecting will not provide significant incentives for conservation of biodiversity.

The conclusions of the Simpson study rest on a number of assumptions. First, the investigators' marginal analysis implies that high-quality samples of every higher plant species are readily and continuously available to pharmaceutical researchers. The researchers also assume that discovery of ten new pharmaceutical products per year would saturate the potential demand for new pharmaceutical products. In addition, they assume that discovery of a new drug in one therapeutic area does not affect the demand for other types of new drugs.

While the marginal value of higher plant samples to the pharmaceutical industry may be a declining function, the marginal cost of supplying samples of all species of higher plants is an increasing function. The equilibrium supply of plant samples will therefore be significantly less than the total number of species, creating the potential for greater conservation incentives than the study would indicate. In addition, while the number of new drug approvals by the Food and Drug Administration (FDA) has averaged approximately ten per year, it is incorrect to assume, as do Simpson and colleagues, that this rate of new drug approval is equivalent to the potential demand for new pharmaceutical products.[2] Also questionable is their assumption that the demand for new pharmaceutical products in one therapeutic area will not be affected by the discovery of other types of drugs. It would be reasonable to expect the demand for new arthritis and anticancer drugs to increase as a result of the discovery of other drugs that extend life expectancy.

The principal objective of each of the studies discussed above was to estimate the value of preserving a species or natural area for pharmaceutical research. None of these studies was intended to provide insights into how to manage a biochemical prospecting program to maximize net benefits either to the organization conducting the research or to society in general. As a result, these studies tend to model the pharmaceutical R&D process as a black box. Costs and success rate estimates for developing a new drug from biological material are treated as if they are indivisible rather than occurring in stages with decision points and new information available at each stage. In addition, biological samples and extracts are modeled as uniform commodities that are not distinguished by the quality of the information associated with them. Finally, none of these studies incorporates into their models any analysis of how the development of new biotechnologies and the continued emergence of drug-resistant diseases would affect pharmaceutical R&D decisions or the option value of preserving a species for pharmaceutical research.

To provide practical guidance to companies, countries, and international organizations that have an interest in the emerging biochemical prospecting market, it is necessary to develop more detailed and flexible models of natural product research in the pharmaceutical industry. It is also essential to refine the analysis of how the pharmaceutical value of biodiversity should be incorporated into conservation and development plans of source countries. A more systematic analysis of the political economy of this emerging market is also needed to guide international policy development.

THE NATURAL PRODUCT RESEARCH PROCESS
IN THE PHARMACEUTICAL INDUSTRY

A biochemical prospecting effort begins with the development of an appropriate strategy for the collection of biological samples. The collection process may be random, but often it is guided by biomedical, ethnological, or ecological knowledge. A particular species of plant or animal may concentrate different compounds in particular parts or organs of its body. The chemical structure of the organism may change at different times of the year or may vary over the life cycle of the organism. Different soil conditions, food sources, or intraspecies genetic variations can also lead to significant chemical differences between subpopulations or individuals of the same species. Consequently, it is always desirable to obtain additional supplies of any sample of interest from the same location, subpopulation, or individual as the original sample. No matter what strategy is used to select samples for testing, detailed information must be maintained about the biological source, geographic location, time of collection, and environmental conditions of each sample.

Once the collection of biological samples is under way, each extract prepared from these samples is subjected to one or more screening procedures to determine its ability to inhibit or stimulate certain biological activities associated with particular diseases or healing processes. The extracts that display the most activity in the first stage of tests are fractionated and put through another set of tests. Through the use of a variety of automated bioassays, thousands of biological extracts can be quickly screened in this fashion, although only a few are likely to exhibit therapeutically useful levels of chemical activity. In a process known as "dereplication," these few promising extracts will then be analyzed more fully to isolate chemically active compounds and determine whether they are truly novel or have been previously discovered.

Occasionally, a biochemical prospecting effort will provide pharmaceutical companies with the active ingredient for a new prescription medicine with little or no modification to the original natural product. More frequently, however, novel biological compounds provide the prospecting organization with a lead, i.e., some insight into the chemical structure of compounds that have the desired therapeutic effects. At several stages in the drug development process, a biologically derived lead is likely to be chemically modified in an effort to enhance the compound's therapeutic value or to eliminate some of its side effects. Once a potentially valuable compound has been isolated from a biological extract and its chemical composition determined, subsequent stages of the R&D process are essentially the same as those for a compound that was synthesized in the laboratory, with the obvious exception that it may eventually become necessary or desirable to synthesize the biologically derived lead.

After screening, chemical isolation, and dereplication, the next phase of the drug development process normally consists of a series of tests involving animal subjects. Additional in vitro tests may also be performed at this time. The objectives of this preclinical phase are to estimate the effective and toxic dose ranges for the compound and to determine its pharmacological effects and toxicity symptoms. If the preclinical tests provide evidence that the original or modified compound may be relatively efficacious and safe in treating certain diseases as compared to other available drugs, then a request is made to the FDA and/or its regulatory counterpart in other countries to begin clinical human testing.

In the United States, the request to begin human testing takes the form of an application for the investigation of a new drug (IND). The clinical or IND phase involves three sets of human tests designed to evaluate toxicity, therapeutic value, and unanticipated side effects. Normally, long-term animal studies will be conducted simultaneously with the clinical trials to provide an indication of any deleterious effects over longer periods of use. If the clinical testing phase provides sufficient evidence that the new drug is effective and safe, a new drug application (NDA) will be submitted for regulatory approval. Approval of the NDA is considered the benchmark of a technically successful R&D process. The major steps in the development of a new drug from biological source material are summarized in Figure 1.1. The entire process from collection of compounds to NDA approval can take ten years or more to complete (FDA 1988).

Simultaneous with this technical development process is an ongoing effort to evaluate and plan the commercial aspects involved in the

FIGURE 1.1. Biochemical Prospecting and the Drug Development Process

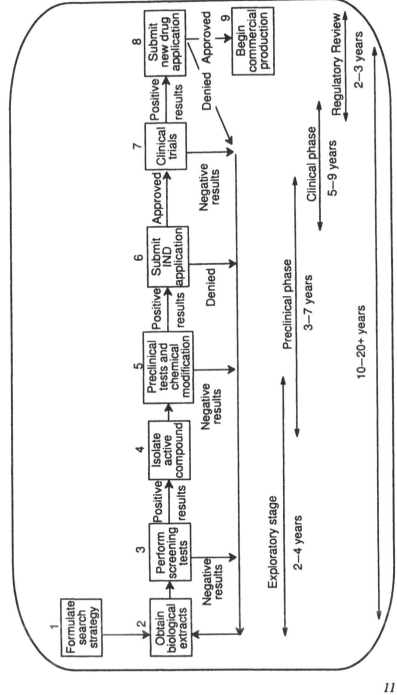

introduction of a new drug. The successful introduction of any new product requires market research, profitability analysis, production planning, marketing, and distribution. The revenues that are expected to be generated by a new drug must be assessed in relation to the probability and potential costs of developing it. Many promising new chemical entities may not proceed past the exploratory or preclinical phases due to other research priorities, market conditions, public opinion, or regulatory considerations. Commercial, institutional, and social factors must therefore be considered as integral parts of the drug development process.

PROSPECTING STRATEGIES

Biochemical prospecting strategies can be broadly grouped into four general categories: random, biomedical, ethnobotanical, and ecological. The strategy or set of strategies to be employed will depend on the therapeutic targets of the prospecting effort, the ecological and cultural characteristics of the regions to be searched, the results of prior natural product research programs, and the research capabilities of the organizations involved. In the process of screening and analyzing biological extracts, the novel chemical structure of a particular compound or its unanticipated side effects may occasionally provide insights into the source or characteristics of new drugs that are unrelated to the focus of the prospecting effort. A well-designed biochemical prospecting program will therefore build in some flexibility to pursue new leads and to respond to unanticipated discoveries.

Random Search Processes

A random search process will usually result in a relatively low success rate per extract tested. However, as screening techniques for certain types of diseases have become more rapid and less expensive, random or comprehensive searches have become more practical. In particular, a random search strategy is often most appropriate when very few leads exist regarding the chemical characteristics of compounds that could be effective against the target disease. Rapid screening of a broad range of biological extracts might yield results that provide a basis for subsequent, more focused natural product screening and rational drug design efforts.

Using Taxonomic and Biomedical Information in the Search Process

A more focused search strategy might begin with the knowledge that existing drugs for certain diseases were developed from a particular class of plants, animal, or bacteria. In this case, extracts from genetically similar organisms would be sought for screening and analysis. For example, the discovery of penicillin prompted researchers to test thousands of mold and bacteria species, which eventually led to the development of many new antibiotics (Oldfield 1984, p. 122). More recently, a British firm, Xenova Ltd., has assembled a collection of over 20,000 fungi and microorganisms on which it is prepared to perform a wide range of screening tests on a contractual basis for other corporations or research institutes (Pollock 1992).

Extracts might also be sought from genetically diverse species that are thought to produce chemical compounds similar in structure to an effective existing drug. A biochemically directed prospecting effort of this kind occurred after the Mexican government tried to control the price of diosgenin, an extract of Mexican yams (dioscorea), from which the vast majority of steroids were manufactured during the 1970s. The search for alternative presteroidal compounds led to the development of biological and chemical processes that can use several other types of plant material as inputs in the manufacture of steroids, notably soybeans and the West African Calabar bean (Myers 1992, p. 218).

If the search is being guided by biochemical information obtained from an existing drug, the screening tests might be calibrated to identify only very high levels of chemical activity. However, if effective drugs for a disease or group of diseases have not yet been developed, the tests utilized to screen new compounds might be calibrated to detect much lower levels of activity.

Relative to a random search strategy, a biomedically focused search can be more rapid, be less expensive, and have a higher probability of yielding biological extracts that display the desired chemical properties. Unfortunately, a biomedically based search strategy is only possible when there are some clues regarding the types of compounds likely to be effective against the target disease(s). Even then there is a risk that no new information will be gained as a result of the search process. For instance, an overly focused search might yield a relatively high percentage of active compounds, all of which prove to be virtually identical to the existing drug that provided the original search criteria.

Ethnobiological Search Strategies

Biomedical prospecting strategies based upon the chemical structure of existing drugs or knowledge of the chemical characteristics of disease organisms draw upon the knowledge base developed by one particular culture, modern technological society. Biochemical prospecting strategies based upon ethnobiological information would expand the source of information to include the knowledge and practices of a broader range of cultures. Shaman Pharmaceuticals is a start-up company that has concentrated its drug discovery efforts exclusively on ethnobiological leads (King and Tempesta 1993). Several of the biochemical prospecting efforts supported through the NIH's International Cooperative Biodiversity group (ICBG) program also include an ethnobiological approach for selecting samples to screen (Grifo et al. 1996).

In the first stage of an ethnobiologically based prospecting effort, the specific plant or animal extracts used by indigenous healers might be tested for commercially promising chemical properties. A second stage might involve isolating the effective chemical compound and expanding the search to include other species known to produce similar compounds.

One of the obvious strengths of the ethnobiological search strategy is that, at least within a given culture, the plants and animals that are selected for screening are known to produce compounds with significant therapeutic or toxicological effects. The probability of isolating highly active chemical compounds from any given extract would therefore be greater than a random search strategy. Of course, ethnobiologically based prospecting processes would still include efforts to alter the chemical structure of any biologically derived leads to increase their effectiveness or to reduce their toxicity.

Although the probability of obtaining chemically active compounds may be increased through the use of an ethnobiological search process, it may be difficult to focus the search on a specific therapeutic objective. Traditional pharmacopoeias may not include treatments specifically targeted to certain modern ailments such as heart disease, cancer, or AIDS. Some biological extracts utilized by indigenous healers could ultimately provide leads to effective drugs for these or other diseases that were not the original targets of the indigenous remedies, but it is often difficult to anticipate this in advance. The rosy periwinkle (catharanthus plant), for instance, was first investigated in response to reports that its leaves were used as a traditional remedy for diabetes (Tyler, Lynn, and Robbers 1988, p. 17). Similarly, the cardiovascular benefits of quinine were only discovered when malaria patients treated with quinine were found to be free of cardiac arrhythmias (Oldfield 1984, p. 107)

Ecologically Informed Search Strategies

Just as ethnobiological knowledge can be defined as including modern biomedical information, an ecologically based search strategy can be viewed as encompassing the ethnobiological approach in the sense that ecological interactions reflect the biochemical "knowledge" of all species, not just Homo sapiens. Compounds released by certain plants under certain conditions can effectively repel normally voracious insects. Diseased animals are often observed to alter their foraging habits to include certain plants with medicinal properties. Many predator-prey, parasite-host, and herbivore-plant relationships have been found to involve a kind of "chemical arms race," while the many elaborate, symbiotic relationships found between rainforest species can also provide evidence of chemical compounds worth investigating (Kricher 1989, pp. 180–210). Knowledge of the chemical interactions between species can provide important leads for the biochemical prospecting process. One of the first large-scale efforts to test the efficacy of ecological information in a drug discovery program is being conducted in the arid tropical forest of Costa Rica's Guanacaste National Park as part of a collaboration among Cornell University, INBio, and Bristol-Myers Squibb, with support from the ICBG program.

As with biomedically or ethnobiologically informed search strategies, an ecologically based approach can reduce the number of species that must be investigated and minimize the number of tests required to discover and isolate useful compounds. For instance, Cor Therapeutics of South San Francisco is testing a drug to prevent unwanted blood clots. The drug was reportedly developed after screening the venom of only 70 species of snakes (Pollock 1992). It may not always be possible, however, to focus an ecologically based prospecting effort on a treatment for a particular disease or commercial product. An ecological search will of necessity be limited to those species for which information exists regarding their chemical ecology. Of course, the prospecting process itself may involve collecting new ecological information as a means of generating leads. However, the added cost and time of gathering ecological information that may be valuable for purposes of biochemical prospecting must be taken into account in evaluating the merits of such an endeavor.

SELECTING A PROSPECTING STRATEGY

Each of the search strategies outlined above has certain strengths and weaknesses. The most important tradeoff is between a more focused search with higher probabilities of discovering chemically active compounds and a reduced pool of species from which to collect extracts. In addition, the random and biomedically driven search strategies can more readily incorporate a particular therapeutic objective as the focus of the search. An ethnobiologically or ecologically based search process may need to be more open to investigating a wider range of potential uses for the extracts collected. The strategy or combination of search strategies most appropriate will depend on the objectives of the search; the scientific capabilities of the firm(s) or research institution(s) engaged in the prospecting effort; the types of species present within the target ecosystem; and the ecological knowledge, specimen collection, and support services that are available. Most large-scale biochemical prospecting efforts, such as the NCI's natural products screening program or the projects supported through the ICBG program, are likely to involve the cooperation of several organizations and to incorporate biochemical information, ethnomedicinal leads, and insights gleaned from ecological interactions, as well as more comprehensive screening of biological extracts that are readily available.

BIOCHEMICAL PROSPECTING AND OTHER METHODS OF DRUG DISCOVERY

Natural product research within the pharmaceutical industry is often considered to be a cyclical process, with periods of high interest and investment followed by periods of inactivity. These cyclical swings may be triggered by a new drug discovery or lack thereof, but ultimately, they are attributable to perceived changes in the economics of natural product research relative to other forms of drug discovery. The development of automated, high-throughput screening technologies has helped to keep more comprehensive biological screening programs competitive with rational drug design efforts (Armond 1994). However, these same screening technologies, together with more rapid techniques for synthesizing and modifying certain classes of molecules, have also reduced the cost of a new approach to drug discovery based on combinatorial chemical synthesis (Houghten 1988; Harris 1995).

Drug screening programs based on combinatorial chemistry have several important advantages. First, millions of new molecules can be synthesized rapidly and inexpensively. In addition, the chemical structure of any molecule that shows high levels of activity in preliminary screening tests can usually be readily determined, synthesized in large quantities, and easily modified for further testing. This contrasts with natural product screening programs, where it may be difficult to isolate and characterize the active compounds in any extracts that test positively. Moreover, once the chemical structure of an active natural product has been determined, there is no guarantee that it can be easily synthesized or modified. Soejarto and Farnsworth (1989) estimate that less than 5 percent of natural product medicines are commercially produced by chemical synthesis.

The disadvantages of natural product research are also the source of its principal strength, which is the tremendous diversity of chemical compounds found in nature (Devlin 1995). The goal of drug discovery is to identify molecules having properties that can inhibit a disease or activate a healing response. If we think of exploring a multidimensional "space," where each dimension represents the possible range of a relevant chemical characteristic, molecules with the desired therapeutic properties are likely to occupy a very small portion of this space. In some cases, sufficient biochemical information about the receptor enzyme or disease organism is available to identify a potential mechanism of action for an effective new drug. Given this information, the researcher can pursue a rational drug design effort because he or she has some understanding of where in this molecular space a new drug might be found. For many diseases and ailments, unfortunately, this type of information is simply not available. The mechanism of action by which aspirin relieves pain has only recently been discovered, even though aspirin has been marketed as a drug for almost 100 years (Loll, Picot, and Garavito 1995). In situations where the mechanism of action or even the target receptor is not well-understood, access to a diverse array of biologically derived molecules can be particularly valuable.

Consider a three-dimensional molecular space where each axis defines a molecular characteristic of relevance to a proposed new drug discovery effort. The screening test that will be used in this drug discovery effort can detect bioactivity of molecules that lie within a certain distance in each "direction" from the point in molecular space occupied by the assay. Libraries of synthetically derived compounds are often close analogues of each other (Harris 1995). In the context of our spatial analogy, they would be tightly grouped in one small region of the molecular space of interest. As shown in the left side of Figure 1.2, the ideal new drug may be represented by a combination of characteristics that is quite distant from the region in molecular space where the synthetic compounds are grouped. If this is the case, it is entirely possible that none of the synthetically developed compounds will react strongly with the bioassay, and little new information will be obtained about the structure of an effective new drug.

Now consider a screening program involving a collection of biological extracts drawn from widely divergent taxonomic groups, ecological niches, and geographic regions. Each of these extracts may contain hundreds or thousands of different molecules, and the total molecular diversity embodied in the entire collection of

FIGURE 1.2. Exploring Molecular Space

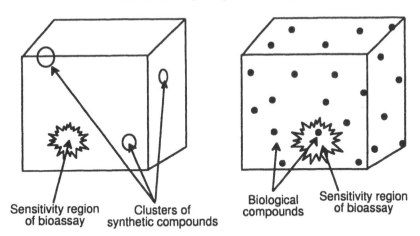

Sensitivity region   Clusters of   Biological   Sensitivity region
of bioassay   synthetic compounds compounds   of bioassay

extracts is likely to be quite high. If the molecules are distributed randomly throughout the molecular space of interest, as shown on the right side of Figure 1.2, then testing the entire collection of extracts is likely to identify one or more extracts that react strongly with the screen. After the active compound in these extracts is isolated, the prospecting organization can derive important new information about the structure of molecules that are likely to be effective in the therapeutic area under investigation.

The spatial analogy outlined above highlights the importance of obtaining a highly diverse supply of molecules to screen. It also indicates the potential synergy between natural product research and other forms of drug discovery. By isolating and analyzing the structure of molecules that react with a bioassay, it is possible to determine what area of molecular space to search in more detail, i.e., what types of analog molecules should be developed and evaluated in subsequent tests. There are some indications that it may soon be possible to use molecular replication techniques to develop analogs from a broader set of biologically derived molecules (Rubeck 1994; Joyce 1992). If the chemical and biotechnological techniques can be refined to the point where analogs of almost any molecule can be generated rapidly and inexpensively, then the tremendous diversity of biologically derived molecules can be fully exploited.

Chapter 2

A Model of the Biochemical Prospecting Process

INTRODUCTION

Pharmaceutical R&D can be viewed as a series of lotteries that require substantial expenditures and yield uncertain returns a decade or more in the future. In most cases, it is necessary to screen thousands of synthetically developed or biologically derived compounds to obtain a few that are promising enough to warrant preclinical animal trials (Burger 1990). Developing or obtaining these compounds and screening them for a particular set of chemical reactions can take several years. Of those few compounds that show some promise after initial screening, as few as one out of ten may advance through preclinical and clinical testing to eventually receive regulatory approval (Balthasar, Boschi, and Menke 1978; Hansen 1979; FDA 1988; DiMasi et al. 1991). These preclinical and clinical trials can take more than 10 years to complete and require expenditures of $100 million or more, not including financing costs. Regulatory review of new drug applications requires two to three more years. Once a new drug is approved, revenues can be expected to rise over the first few years, remain relatively steady until patent protection expires, and then ultimately decline due to competition from generic drugs or new products (Statman 1983; Grabowski and Vernon 1990).

The decision theoretic models of the pharmaceutical R&D process developed in this chapter can be used to evaluate many of the critical choices faced by a biochemical prospecting organization.[1] After presenting the equations that constitute the basic model, I will illustrate some of its potential applications using plausible estimates for essential data inputs. I will also outline a more complex version of the basic model, highlighting the similarity between pharmaceutical R&D and a sequence of call options. Finally, I will discuss how the models could be employed to determine the optimum number of samples to obtain for screening and when to terminate a screening program.

THE BASIC MODEL

The basic conceptual framework outlined below for determining the expected cost of pharmaceutical R&D is similar to the approach used in studies by Hansen (1979) and DiMasi and colleagues (1991). However, while these other studies have attempted to estimate the ex-post cost of developing a new drug, I have developed an ex-ante model to estimate the net present value of proceeding with pharmaceutical R&D, given a specified quantity of biological extracts or synthetically derived compounds.

Expected Present Value of R&D Costs

Let N be the number of extracts originally obtained for primary screening, let M be the number of different therapeutic indicators included in the primary screening phase, let s_1 be the average success rate of crude extracts in each type of primary screening test, let s_j be the conditional success rate in phase j (given positive test results in the previous phase), let FC_i be the fixed cost of phase i, and let c_i be the variable cost in phase i of screening or analyzing each extract or compound that tested positively in the previous phase. Then the expected cost of phase i, (EC_i), can be defined as follows:

$$EC_i = FC_i + NMc_i \prod_{j=0}^{i-1} s_j \qquad (2.1)$$

where $s_o = 1$.

If we assume that expenditures occur evenly throughout each R&D phase, then the present value expected cost of phase i $(PVEC_i)$ can be estimated as follows:

$$PVEC_i = \left(\frac{EC_i}{d_i}\right) \sum_{t=0}^{d_i-1} (1+\delta) - (t + D_{i-1}) \qquad (2.2)$$

Where d_i is the expected duration of phase i, in years, and δ is the effective annual discount rate and,

$$D_i = \sum_{j=1}^{i} d_j \qquad (2.2a)$$

is the total duration in years of all phases up to and including phase i.

If the prospecting organization is a profitable private company, the costs of pharmaceutical R&D can be deducted from before-tax net revenues, thereby providing a tax benefit. If τ is the effective corporate tax rate, the present value of the expected cost of phase i, net of the tax deduction, is simply $(1-\tau)(PVEC_i)$.

If there are n phases in the pharmaceutical R&D process, then the present value of expected total costs is simply the sum of the present values of the expected cost of each phase, as shown in Equation 2.3.

$$PVETC = \sum_{i=1}^{n} [PVEC_i] = \sum_{i=1}^{n} \left(\frac{EC_i}{d_i}\right) \sum_{t=0}^{d_i-1} (1+\delta) - t - D_{i-1} \qquad (2.3)$$

Similarly, the present value of expected total costs, net of tax benefits, is $(1-\tau)(PVETC)$.

Present Value of Expected Benefits

The present value of expected revenues to be derived from obtaining N biological extracts is a function of the number of approved new drugs that can be expected to result from R&D efforts utilizing these extracts, the timing and magnitude of anticipated revenues of each new drug net of manufacturing and marketing costs, and the discount rate.

If the prospecting organization plans to screen N natural compounds for M different therapeutic indicators, and new therapeutic targets can be substituted if several promising leads are discovered for any of the original ones, then the expected number of new drugs receiving regulatory approval (A), can be estimated by multiplying the product of M and N by the probability of any given compound advancing through all phases of the R&D process.

$$A = NM \prod_{i=1}^{n} s_i \qquad (2.4)$$

At the start of the prospecting process, the present value of expected before-tax gross revenues $(PVEGR)$ is the expected number of newly approved drugs (A) multiplied by the discounted value of the expected before-tax annual revenues of a new drug, as shown here:[2]

$$PVEGR = A \sum_{t=1}^{D_n+T} R_t (1+\delta)^{-t} \qquad (2.5)$$

where R_t is the expected gross revenue derived from a new drug in year t after the start of research and development, and T is the average commercial life of a new drug in years.

In addition to R&D, an organization that develops and markets a new drug would incur expenses for production plant and equipment, marketing, operations, and administrative overhead. To account for these costs, I shall define the contribution margin (q) as the average proportion of annual revenues available after deducting all production and operating costs other than R&D. Let Z_t be the cost in year t of any initial capital and marketing expenses not accounted for by q. Then the present value of expected before-tax revenues, net of all costs except R&D, can be computed as follows:

$$PVENR = qA \sum_{t=1}^{D_n+T} (R_t - Z_t)(1+\delta)^{-t} \qquad (2.6)$$

After-tax net revenues would simply be $(1 - r)PVENR$.

If the prospecting organization is a public research institution, such as the National Cancer Institute, or, for purposes of policy analysis, one is simply concerned with estimating the social rather than private benefits of a prospecting endeavor, then taxes should not be considered at all, and benefits would have to include not only net revenues but also the value of a new drug to consumers, in excess of its market price, as well as any additional benefits to society (e.g., through reduced contagion or increased productivity). I shall represent the value of any consumer surplus and additional social benefits as a multiplier (*m*) of the drug's net revenues. The expected benefits to society from marketing an effective new drug would therefore be:

$$PVEB = (M)(PVENR) \qquad (2.7)$$

where the discount rate being used to compute present values represents the full opportunity costs to society of devoting resources to the biochemical prospecting endeavor.[3]

Expected Net Present Value

For a private prospecting organization, the expected net present value of obtaining *N* biological extracts is computed by subtracting the present value of expected R&D costs, net of tax benefits, from the after-tax present value of net revenues, as shown below:

$$ENPV_{priv} = (1 - r)(PVENR - PVETC) \qquad (2.8)$$

The expected net present value to society can be computed by utilizing a discount rate that incorporates the full opportunity costs of investments in pharmaceutical R&D and subtracting the present value of expected R&D costs from the expected present value of social benefits as shown below:

$$ENPV_{(soc)} = m(PVENR) - PVETC \qquad (2.9)$$

A Graphical Representation of the Model

It is possible to depict the costs, risks, and potential payoffs from the pharmaceutical R&D process graphically in the form of a decision tree, as shown in Figure 2.1. Depicting the R&D process as a decision tree can serve to clarify the choices available to the prospecting organization and to highlight the increasing value of an individual biological extract or isolated chemical compound as it

FIGURE 2.1. Decision Tree for Biochemical Prospecting Opportunity

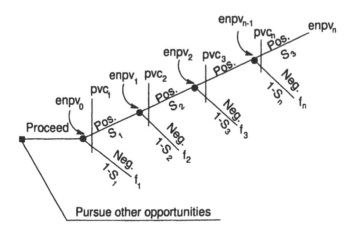

proceeds through each stage of the R&D process. Understanding the biochemical prospecting and R&D process as a series of decisions is also helpful in evaluating alternative prospecting strategies and contractual arrangements.

To utilize a decision tree to calculate the value of an extract at any point in the R&D process, it is necessary to follow a procedure known as averaging out and folding back. Assume that there are n phases in the R&D process and that $enpv_n$ is the present value of net benefits expected to be received after successful completion of the final phase (i.e., the expected net benefits associated with receiving regulatory approval to market a new drug).[4] Let f_n be the expected benefits, if any, associated with failure or negative results in the final phase.[5] Let s_n be the probability of successful results in phase n, conditional on a compound having proceeded through the R&D process to reach the final phase. The conditional probability of failure in the final phase would therefore be $1 - s_n$. Finally, let pvc_n be the present value of the cost of proceeding with the final phase. After successful completion of phase $n - 1$, the expected net benefit of proceeding with phase n is therefore

$$enpv_{n-1} = (s_n)(enpv_n) + (1-s_n)(f_n) - pvc_n \qquad (2.10)$$

Similarly, after successful completion of phase $n*2$, the expected benefit of proceeding with phase $n-1$, is:

$$enpv_{n-2} = (s_{n-1})(enpv_{n-1})+(1-s_{n-1})(f_{n-1})-pvc_{n-1}$$

(2.11)

This process of moving back through the decision tree can be continually repeated to generate the expected value of obtaining an unscreened biological extract. The recursive form of Equation 2.10, which can be used to calculate the expected benefit at the end of any phase, is shown below:

$$enpv_i = enpv_n \prod_{j=i+1}^{n}(s_j) + \sum_{j=i+1}^{n}[(1-s_j)f_j-pvc_j]\prod_{k=i}^{j-1}(s_k)$$

(2.12)

where $s_i = 1$.

If the analysis is being performed from the point of view of a private prospecting organization at the start of the R&D process, the potential benefits at the end of the decision tree ($enpv_n$) would be the after-tax present value of expected revenues, net of all expenses except R&D. This is equivalent to $(1 - r)PVNER$ computed from Equation 2.6, where A, the number of new drugs receiving regulatory approval, is equal to one. If the prospecting organization is a public entity, then $enpv_n$ would be equal to *PVEB* as defined in Equation 2.7.

When evaluated at $i = 0$, Equation 2.12 yields the expected net present value of obtaining one biological extract for evaluation in relation to one therapeutic target. If $f_j = 0$ for all j, Equation 2.12 yields values identical to those of Equations 2.8 and 2.9, for private and public prospecting organizations respectively, where N, the number of compounds obtained for testing, and M, the number of independent primary screening tests, are both equal to one.

Equation 2.12 can also be utilized to calculate the expected value of an extract or compound that has advanced through one or more stages of the R&D process. However, in this regard it is important to be clear about the temporal perspective of the valuation process. Given a supply of crude extracts, the prospecting organization would be interested in the expected present value of proceeding with the primary screening phase. Therefore, all expected costs and benefits should be discounted back to the start of the R&D process.

However, if a prospecting organization has ten compounds that have successfully proceeded through the third phase of the R&D process, and it wishes to compute the expected net present value of proceeding to Phase IV for each compound, then all expected costs and benefits should be discounted to the start of Phase IV, rather than back to the start of Phase I. Analysis of the increasing value of a compound as it proceeds through the R&D process will be discussed in more detail in subsequent chapters.

DEFINING THE R&D PROCESS

As outlined in the previous chapter, the pharmaceutical R&D process is often divided into six basic phases: exploratory research, preclinical trials, three phases of clinical trials, and regulatory review of a new drug application (NDA). In addition, long-term animal studies are often conducted simultaneously with clinical testing to evaluate any chronic effects of a new drug. Although the study by DiMasi and colleagues provides empirical data on the costs and duration of the clinical phases of pharmaceutical R&D, it does not provide a similar level of detail for earlier phases of the R&D process. Since it is very difficult for a pharmaceutical company to associate the costs of a diverse exploratory research program with the eventual regulatory approval of a particular drug or set of drugs, exploratory and preclinical R&D costs have often been estimated simply as a multiple of clinical testing costs.[6]

To analyze the economic benefits of securing a supply of biologically derived compounds, I have divided the exploratory research stage into four phases and incorporated separate estimates of the costs and success rates for each of these phases as well as for preclinical animal testing. This detailed view of the early phases of the R&D process permits more meaningful analysis of alternative prospecting strategies and contract terms. It also permits additional information on the actual costs and success probabilities of biochemical prospecting efforts to be readily incorporated into the analysis.

The first phase of exploratory research is defined to include the collection, preparation, and initial screening of biological extracts. The second phase consists of secondary screening intended to verify preliminary test results. Any extract with positive test results in primary and secondary screening is then analyzed to determine if the active compound is a new chemical entity that has not been previously discovered. This process, known as isolation and dereplication, has been incorporated into the third phase of exploratory research together with preliminary toxicological evaluation. The fourth phase of exploratory research would involve efforts to synthesize, modify, or combine attributes of those novel compounds that had demonstrated positive test results in preliminary screening and toxicological evaluation. In some cases, compounds that showed promise in exploratory research would still proceed to preclinical animal testing even if chemical synthesis had not been achieved. Vincristine, derived from the rosy periwinkle, and taxol, derived from the Pacific yew, are two examples of drugs that were marketed before economical methods of chemical synthesis had been developed. However, depending on the potential market for the drug candidate, prospecting organizations may be reluctant to proceed with costly preclinical and clinical trials if a commercial supply of the compound cannot be assured either through economical synthesis or large-scale production from the source species.

SOME COMPLICATIONS TO THE BASIC MODEL

As screening of a large quantity of extracts proceeds, there is an increasing probability that extracts which test positively, will turn out to contain only compounds that have been previously isolated and characterized. Consequently, the percentage of compounds proceeding past chemical isolation and dereplication into subsequent R&D phases would be expected to decrease as the number of compounds already screened increases.

The percentage of "hits" that turn out to contain only previously discovered compounds will depend on several factors. Most important is whether certain ubiquitous bioactive compounds, such as tannins, are removed in prior stages either through extraction or selective screening tests. If this is not the case, the isolation and dereplication phase can be thought of as a two-stage process. The first stage of the dereplication process would have a high failure rate due to elimination of extracts containing only common bioactive compounds. Extracts or isolated compounds that had proceeded through this first stage of dereplication would presumably have a much lower failure rate in the second stage of dereplication because the focus there would be on whether these comparatively rare compounds had been discovered in prior natural product research programs.

This raises the second factor affecting the dereplication rate: the degree of natural product research that has already been conducted in relation to the biological subject matter and the therapeutic targets that are the focus of the biochemical prospecting effort. The more already conducted research there is, the more likely it is that even relatively rare compounds have been previously discovered and investigated. Still, even if substantial biological screening has been conducted on the same species in the therapeutic areas of interest, it is important to consider whether the bioassays currently being used are expected to react with compounds that would have been missed in previous biological screening efforts.

The characteristics of the extracts that will be screened must also be considered. If the extracts are all drawn from similar species, then as screening continues, many of the same compounds are likely to be identified again and again. However, if the extracts to be screened will be drawn from a more taxonomically diverse group of species, discovery of one or more novel compounds may not significantly reduce the possibility of discovering other novel compounds in the species yet to be screened.

The relationship between the success rate of an extract in the dereplication phase and the number of extracts previously screened is likely to differ for various types of screening programs. Unfortunately, data from which to estimate this relationship is not readily available. For purposes of sensitivity analysis, I shall use the following functional relationship, which is flexible enough to incorporate the considerations outlined:

$$s_{d,k} = \left[(1-r)^{1+\sum_{j=0}^{i-1} s_j} + r(1-s_{d,0})^k \right] s_{d,0} \qquad (2.13)$$

where $s_{d,k}$ is the success rate of the kth compound in the dereplication phase, $s_{d,0}$ is the initial success rate that would be dependent on the novelty of the preliminary screening assays and the amount of previous natural product research in this area, and r is a factor from 0 to 1, with a value of 0 indicating no expected chemical replication between extracts entering the dereplication phase and a value of one indicating complete replication, i.e., identical extracts. The value of r in Equation 2.13 should be an estimate of the probability of repeated discovery of a new compound. It should not include any consideration of replication of common compounds or chemicals discovered in previous screening programs, which is already accounted for through the estimated value of $s_{d,0}$. For screening programs involving thousands of biological extracts, the declining success rate of the dereplication phase shown in Equation 2.13 should be incorporated into Equations 2.1 and 2.4, which are used to estimate R&D costs and new product revenues, respectively.

The simple linear relationship presented in Equation 2.4 also assumes that if a new drug is successfully developed, or a number of highly promising leads discovered, for one therapeutic target, then the prospecting organization will keep the number of unsatisfied therapeutic objectives constant by substituting new targets in its screening program. If this replacement does not take place, i.e., if development of a new drug reduces the number of therapeutic objectives for which subsequent extracts are screened, then Equation 2.4 should be further modified as follows:

$$A = M \sum_{k=1}^{N} \left(\prod_{j=1}^{n} S_j \right) \left(1 - \prod_{i=1}^{n} S_j \right)^k \qquad (2.14)$$

This modification acknowledges the increasing possibility that a successful new drug will already have been discovered in each therapeutic category as more and more biological extracts are screened.

APPLYING THE MODEL

The following sections summarize available data and a set of assumptions regarding costs, risks, and potential benefits of a representative biochemical prospecting opportunity. Based upon these estimates and assumptions, the net present value of a supply of biological extracts is calculated from the perspectives of a private prospecting organization and a public prospecting organization. Later in this chapter, I will modify these baseline assumptions as part of a general sensitivity analysis. I will also outline several analytical methods for assessing the value of gathering additional information regarding critical parameters of the model.

Determining the Discount Rate

Since the time frame from the start of the prospecting process to the final year of product sales is more than 30 years, the discount rate used to calculate the present value of both costs and revenues is one of the most important factors in the analysis. An appropriate discount rate would reflect the returns available on other investments with similar risks.[7] Based upon the framework of the capital asset pricing model (CAPM), the market cost of capital for investments in a given asset can be estimated from the following equation:

Exp. Return on Equity = Risk-Free Rate + (Beta) x (Market Risk Premium)[8]

For investments in pharmaceutical research and development, the appropriate inputs to the above equation would be the expected rate of return on a risk-free investment of similar time horizon, such as a 30-year treasury bond; the long-term returns, in excess of the risk-free rate, of a well-diversified portfolio of stocks (i.e., the market risk premium); and the expected covariance of returns from pharmaceutical R&D with total market returns (i.e., the asset's beta) over the relevant time period. A common approach to utilizing the CAPM model is to estimate the components of the model from past data.

Estimates of beta for pharmaceutical company stocks range from .96 to 1.06 (Chien and Upson 1980; Statman 1983, p. 82; Grabowski and Vernon 1990).[9] Using a Beta of 1.0 together with Ibbotson and Sinquefeld's (1988) estimates of 1.7 percent as the inflation-adjusted yield on long-term government bonds for the period 1926 to 1987 and 6.8 percent as the long-horizon equity risk premium during this period, the estimated real annual discount rate for pharmaceutical R&D investments would be 1.7 + 6.8 = 8.5 percent. For the more recent ten-year period 1978 to 1987, real riskless returns were 2.62 percent and the long-horizon equity risk premium was 4.27 percent. This yields an estimated real discount rate of 6.89 percent for long-term investments in pharmaceutical companies.

For the baseline analysis, I have used a real annual discount rate of 8.5 percent. In light of more recent data on yields of long-term government bonds and equity risk premiums, this appears to be a conservative assumption.

R&D Costs, Duration, and Success Rates

Many large pharmaceutical companies have installed substantial capacity for screening both biological extracts and synthetic compounds. There is, in fact, a thriving industry, special conferences, and a new professional society devoted to automated high throughput pharmaceutical screening.[10] There are also numerous firms that provide the pharmaceutical industry and nonprofit research institutions with primary screening services. These firms' published prices range from $1,500 to $4,000 per extract or compound, which includes conducting and categorizing the results of primary screening tests for 10 to 35 different therapeutic indicators.

Fixed costs of primary screening will depend on the particular circumstances of the prospecting organization. If the organization has excess screening capacity available or would pay a per extract fee to an independent screening firm, then fixed costs can be ignored. However, if the firm is planning to install new screening equipment for the proposed prospecting activity, then these fixed costs would have to be included in the analysis. For the baseline analysis, I have assumed no fixed costs and an estimate of $100 for the variable cost per extract for each type of primary screening test performed.

Success, or "hit," rates in any preliminary screening program will depend upon the success criteria that have been established for each screening test. In preliminary screening programs involving crude extracts, there is a tradeoff between establishing a lax criteria for success, which increases the probability of isolating novel compounds that are present in only small quantities in the extract but results in increased secondary screening and dereplication costs, and establishing very stringent success criteria, which helps to minimize secondary screening costs but increases the risk of not discovering some potentially valuable compounds. The resolution of this tradeoff involves a combination of subjective judgment and empirical data on the probabilities and relative costs of false positives and false negatives.

Interpretation of available data on natural product screening programs is further complicated by differing definitions of such terms as "hit rate," "active compounds," and "drug leads." With these cautions in mind, I have utilized a success rate of .005 for each primary screening test and a success rate of .40 for secondary screening, based upon data from natural product screening programs (Suffness and Douros 1982; Rosenthal 1995; Thompson 1996; INBio 1992a, 1992b, 1992c; Personal communication with Dr. James McChesney, Department of Pharmacognosy, University of Mississippi, February 3, 1993). These assumptions imply that, on average, 1 out of 500 extracts tested for each therapeutic target will be considered significant enough for the prospecting organization to invest the time and expense involved in chemical isolation and dereplication.

For purposes of the baseline analysis, I have also assumed that the prospecting strategy employs ten primary screens, each testing for a different therapeutic activity, and that collection, preparation, and primary screening of all 15,000 extracts will take 18 months to complete. The baseline analysis also assumes a cost of $1,000 per compound expended over a period of two months for secondary screening and evaluation of results.

I have used an average duration of six months and a cost of $25,000 per extract for the phase of exploratory research that includes chemical isolation, characterization, and dereplication. In the baseline analysis, all compounds entering the isolation and dereplication phase are assumed to have a success probability of 0.10 (i.e., $r = 0$ in Equation 2.13). For the baseline analysis, I have used a value of $r = 0$ in Equation 2.13, indicating that the success rate in the dereplication phase remains constant at 10 percent for all extracts entering the dereplication phase.

After further chemical analysis, modification, and toxicological testing, some novel compounds may be deemed unworthy of further preclinical or clinical trials. In other cases, the prospecting organization might not be able to achieve synthesis or to obtain sufficient quantities of the natural product to continue with preclinical and clinical trials. For the baseline analysis, I have assumed that the prospecting organization is sufficiently dedicated to and prepared for natural product research such that one-half of isolated compounds that successfully proceed through the dereplication phase proceed to preclinical animal trials. The baseline analysis includes a total expenditure of $250,000 per compound for chemical modification, analysis, and toxicological testing during Phase IV of exploratory research.

For preclinical animal testing, I have used an estimate of $771,000 per compound tested.[11] For the preclinical animal testing phase, I have also assumed a duration of one year and that 40 percent of the compounds entering this phase will proceed to clinical testing (Burger 1990, p. 39; Hansen 1979; DiMasi et al. 1991).

The direct costs per trial, success rates, and effective duration of the three phases of clinical trials, as well as long-term toxicity testing in animals, have been derived from the study by DiMasi and colleagues.[12] Table 2.1 summarizes the duration, success probabilities, and expected costs of all phases of the pharmaceutical R&D process for the baseline analysis.

It may be helpful to place the success probabilities outlined in some larger perspective. The product of the assumed success probabilities for the four phases of exploratory research indicates that in each therapeutic category being tested for, 1 candidate for preclinical animal trials will be developed from approximately every 10,000 extracts tested. If this ratio is multiplied by the assumed success probability of the preclinical phase, then in each therapeutic category only 1 compound out of every 25,000 extracts tested can be expected to proceed to the first phase of clinical testing in humans. Burger (1990) indicates that a ratio of 1 compound out of 5,000 is considered to be a conservative estimate of the success rate of general screening procedures up to and including the preclinical phase.

Less than one out of five drug candidates entering clinical trials is assumed to proceed through all clinical phases and receive FDA approval to be marketed as a new drug. Therefore, given the probabilities incorporated into the baseline model, fewer than one out of every 111,000 extracts tested in each therapeutic objective will eventually lead to the development of a new drug. Since the baseline model assumes that extracts are tested for activity in relation to

TABLE 2.1. R&D Costs and Success Rates—Baseline Analysis (in $000s)

# of Extracts Tested	15,000
# of Indicators in Primary Screen	10
Real Discount Rate	8.50%

	Effective Duration (yrs.)	Success Prob. per Trial	Mean # of Successes	Cost per Trial	Pres. Value Cost per Trial	Expected Phase Cost	Pres. Value of Exp. Phase Cost
Initial Screening*	0.75	0.005	750.00	0.10	0.10	15,000	14,548
Secondary Screening	0.10	0.400	300.00	1	1	750	732
Isolation and Dereplication	0.50	0.100	30.00	20	19	6,000	5,712
Synthesis and Modification	1.50	0.500	15.00	250	219	7,500	6,585
Preclinical Trials	1.00	0.400	6.00	771	611	11,570	9,170
Clinical Phase I	1.35	0.750	4.50	3,137	2,259	18,822	13,557
Clinical Phase II**	1.88	0.475	2.14	9,933	6,275	44,698	28,239
Clinical Phase III	2.49	0.700	1.50	18,817	9,956	40,222	21,282
NDA	3.00	0.900	1.35	1,000	423	1,496	633
Cumulative	12.57	0.000009	1.35	33,930	19,765	146,058	100,457

* Cost per trial for this phase is $200 × the number of screening targets.
** Long-term animal testing is included in probabilities and costs of Phase II clinical trials.

ten different therapeutic indicators, approximately 1 out of every 11,000 extracts screened will lead to a new drug. A commonly repeated rule of thumb in the pharmaceutical industry is that approximately 10,000 compounds must be tested to develop one new drug (Balthasar, Boschi, and Menke 1978; PMA 1985; Vagelos 1991). It is unclear, however, whether this industry estimate of overall success probability, or Burger's estimate of preliminary research success rates cited above, refers to random screening programs for numerous therapeutic targets, rational drug design efforts with one therapeutic objective, or some combination of the two.

Expected Revenues

In Grabowski and Vernon's (1990) analysis of 100 new drugs in which the active ingredient was a new chemical entity (NCE) introduced in the United States from 1970 to 1979, audited data were utilized to compile domestic annual hospital and drugstore sales of each NCE through 1986. These historical sales figures were then utilized to extrapolate future revenues of a new drug, based upon a standard 25-year life cycle of drug sales derived from prior studies. In recent years, however, competition from generic drugs and chemically similar follow-up products has reduced the life cycles of newly introduced drugs. To account for this increase in competition, Grabowski and Vernon include some sensitivity analyses in their study using a 20-year product life cycle with a more rapid decline in revenues after patent expiration.

I have utilized a 20-year product life with patent protection and increasing revenues during the first 11 years after product introduction (Vagelos 1991). Revenue estimates during the period of patent protection are based on Grabowski and Vernon's mean sales figures, adjusted for increases in drug prices through 1994.[13] For years 12 through 20 after product introduction, I have assumed a 7.5 percent annual reduction from prior year revenues. No further revenues are assumed after year 20. In the baseline model, I have utilized a multiplier of 1.9 as the ratio of global to U.S. sales of domestically produced pharmaceutical products (Joglekar and Paterson 1986; Grabowski and Vernon 1990). These assumptions yield a slightly lower present value of expected revenues than in Grabowski and Vernon's sensitivity analysis of increased generic competition.

Following Grabowski and Vernon, I have assumed that plant and equipment (P&E) expenditures are equivalent to one-half of gross revenues generated in year 10. Two-thirds of these P&E expenditures occur in the year prior to product launch, with the balance occurring evenly during years 2 through 10. The baseline model also includes initial marketing expenditures equal to 100 percent, 50 percent, and 25 percent of sales in years 1, 2, and 3, respectively. A constant contribution margin (i.e., the proportion of revenues in excess of capital and operating costs other than R&D) of 40 percent is utilized to account for all other administrative and operating costs throughout the life of the product.

Figure 2.2 summarizes the data and assumptions utilized in the baseline model for expected worldwide gross and net revenues derived from each NCE that receives regulatory approval.

The baseline analysis for a private prospecting organization utilizes a tax rate of 35 percent. It is assumed that research and development costs provide a deduction against taxable income in the year in which these expenses are incurred and that all revenues, net of operating, marketing, administrative, and capital expenses, are taxed in the year in which they are received.

Expected Net Present Value

Using a real annual discount rate of 8.5 percent, together with the other assumptions summarized in Table 2.1 and Figure 2.2, the before-tax expected net present value of screening a supply of 15,000 biological extracts for five therapeutic objectives can be computed from Equations 2.3 and 2.6 to be approximately $7.3 million. With a tax rate of 35 percent, the after-tax expected net present value of screening 15,000 biological extracts is $4.7 million. In the baseline analysis, the before-tax expected net present value of screening each extract is simply $4.7 million divided by 15,000, or $487, and the after-tax expected net present value of each extract is approximately $316.[14] These calculations are summarized in Table 2.2.

If the prospecting organization is a government entity, the correct measure of total benefits should include not only the net revenues of

FIGURE 2.2. Expected Present Value of Worldwide Revenues for Each New Drug Baseline Analysis

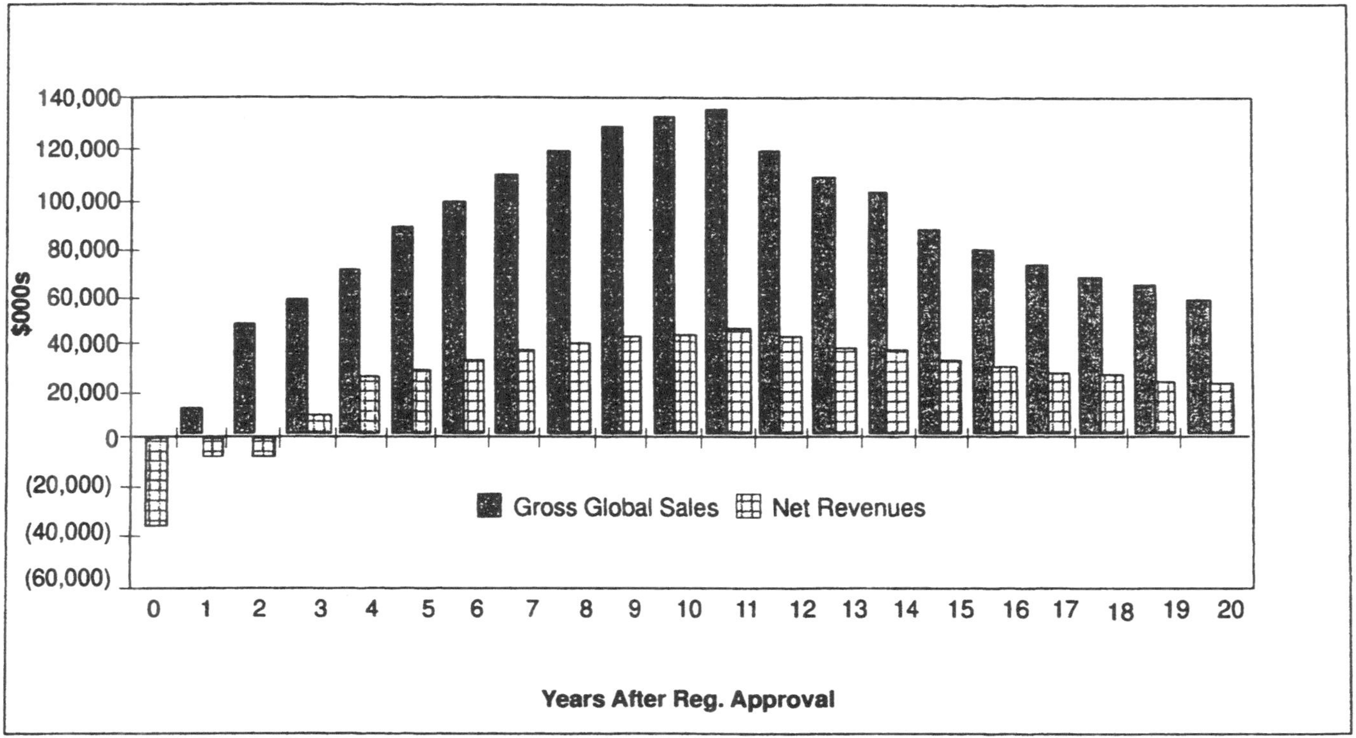

TABLE 2.2. Summary of Present Value Analysis

	Before Tax		After Tax	
	Total	Avg. Per Extract	Total	Avg. Per Extract
PV Exp. Net Revenues	$107,757,315	$7,184	$70,042,255	$4,669
PV Exp. R&D Costs	($100,456,842)	($6,697)	($65,296,947)	($4,353)
Exp. NPV to Priv. Prosp. Org.	$7,300,473	$487	$4,745,308	$316
PV Exp. Net Social Benefits	$115,057,789	$7,671	N/A	N/A
PV Exp. U.S. Net Social Benefits	$12,971,911	$865	N/A	N/A

the originating firm over the patent life of the product but also the profits of generic drug producers after patent protection expires, as well as the additional benefits received by consumers and society in general. One study (Wu 1984) combined data on R&D expenditures, manufacturing and marketing costs, and gross revenues with regression estimates of market demand curves to evaluate private and social rates of return for three new pharmaceutical products. The social benefits from these three pharmaceutical innovations were estimated to be two to four times as large as the revenues received by the innovating firm, net of all costs except R&D.

Given the assumptions in the baseline analysis, a value of 2 for the social benefits multiplier (m) in Equation 2.9, and social opportunity costs represented by a real discount rate of 8.5 percent, the expected present value to society of screening 15,000 extracts is $115 million. This equates to an expected value of $7,671 per extract. If the public prospecting organization were only concerned with the social benefits to U.S. citizens, then the social benefits multiplier should be applied to U.S. rather than worldwide expected net revenues, yielding an estimate of $12.9 million, or approximately $865 per extract, for the present value of U.S. net social benefits.

At this stage, it may be useful to place these expected present values in the context of a hypothetical business or policy decision. The most straightforward interpretation of the results summarized in Table 2.2 is that if a private prospecting organization with the financial and technical capability of developing new drugs from biological source material were to agree with the estimates of costs per trial, success probabilities, and new drug revenues incorporated into the baseline analysis, then, *in the absence of lower cost sources of supply,* that organization should be willing to pay up to $316 for each unscreened biological extract.[15] Similarly, a public prospecting organization sharing the assumptions incorporated into the baseline analysis and interested in maximizing expected worldwide net social benefits should be willing to pay up to $7,671 per extract, *in the absence of less expensive alternative sources of new chemical compounds.* Given the assumptions in the baseline analysis, these are the maximum amounts a private or public prospecting organization should be willing to pay. Competition between suppliers, however, would tend to reduce the market price below these upper limits.

The estimated values of biological extracts assume that the other investment opportunities available to the prospecting organization have an expected real rate of return of 8.5 percent and risk characteristics similar to the hypothetical prospecting program represented in the baseline analysis. In addition, there is an implicit assumption that the benefits of the biochemical prospecting endeavor will be lost or decrease in value if not pursued immediately. This may be the case in a situation involving competition between several profit-seeking firms. If these conditions do not exist and if there is a high degree of technical or economic uncertainty surrounding the prospecting program, the prospecting organization may be able to increase its expected return by waiting to receive, or actively seeking to generate, information that would help resolve this uncertainty (Pindyck 1991). This would reduce the current value of pursuing a large-scale biochemical prospecting opportunity. This option is discussed in more detail later in this chapter.

As discussed previously, evaluation of a biochemical prospecting program can also be depicted in the format of a decision tree. Using the assumptions of the baseline analysis, Figure 2.3 summarizes the calculation of the before-tax expected net present value of screening the first extract for each type of primary screening test. The total before tax *ENPV* of screening the first extract can be computed from Figure 2.3 by multiplying $enpv_0$ by the number of different therapeutic activities being tested for in the primary screening phase.[16] All costs and benefits presented in Figure 2.3 are discounted back to the start of the first phase of the R&D process.

In Figure 2.4, the start of each phase is the temporal point of reference for purposes of discounting expected future costs and benefits. Therefore, in Figure 2.4, the value of a compound at the end of each phase is the maximum amount a prospecting organization should be willing to pay for a compound that has already tested successfully in all R&D phases up to and including that phase but has not yet been tested in any subsequent phases.

Evaluating Prospecting Strategies

A description of various types of prospecting strategies was introduced in the previous chapter, including subjectively random or comprehensive searches involving one or more therapeutic

FIGURE 2.3. Present-Value Analysis of Hypothetical Screening Program Baseline Analysis for Each Screening Objective (all monetary values in $000s)

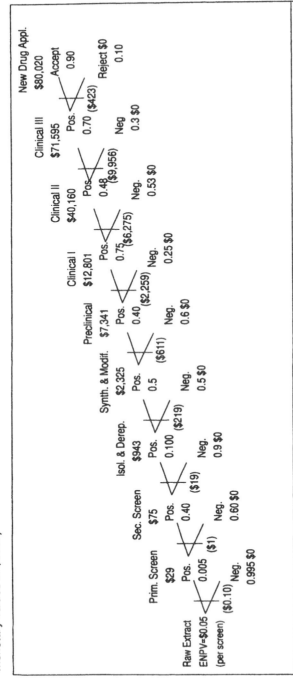

Notes:
1. Figures directly below vertical lines are the present-value cost of testing a compound in that phase.
2. Figures below each outcome indicate conditional probability of occurrence (i.e., success rates for compounds entering the phase).
3. Figures above positive-results branch are the expected present value of compound after successful completion of phase.
4. Value of compound after regulatory approval is the present value of expected revenues from one new drug.
5. Potential costs and revenues are discounted at a real rate of 8.5% based upon effective phase durations presented in Table 2.1.

FIGURE 2.4.Current Value of Compound After Successful Completion of Each Phase Baseline Analysis for Each Screening Objective (all monetary values in $000s)

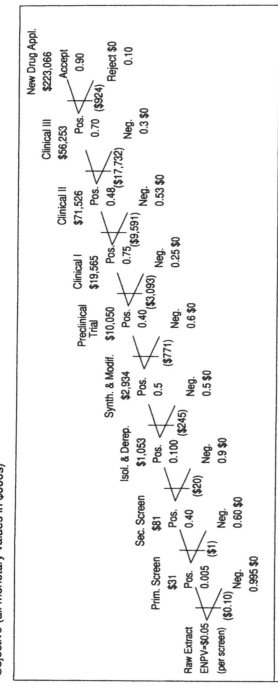

Notes:
1. Figures directly below vertical lines are the costs of testing a compound in that phase, discounted to start of phase.
2. Figures below each outcome indicate conditional probability of occurrence (i.e., success rates for compounds entering the phase).
3. Figures above positive-results branch are the expected current value of compound after successful completion of phase.
4. Value of compound after regulatory approval before-tax value of expected revenues from a new drug discounted to date of approval.
5. Potential costs and revenues are discounted at a real rate of 8.5% based upon effective phase durations presented in Table 2.1.

44

objectives, as well as search strategies that utilize ethnobiological, ecological, or biomedical information to select which species to test. The baseline analysis assumes the prospecting organization is utilizing a subjectively random and objectively comprehensive prospecting strategy. By this I mean that little or no prior information is used to narrow the subject material of the screening program, while the objective of the program is assumed to be the development of one or more new drugs in any of several different therapeutic categories. This assumed prospecting strategy is incorporated into the analysis in the form of a relatively low success probability for each of five different primary screening indicators.

Other prospecting strategies can be modeled by adjusting the number of distinct primary screening tests to be performed, the success probabilities of the primary screening and subsequent exploratory R&D phases, the number of distinct extracts expected to be available given the selection criteria, and any costs involved in determining which species to include in the screening program. If the objective of the prospecting effort involves only a few therapeutic categories in which the estimated market demand for new drugs differs substantially from the average new drug, then the estimates of expected private and public benefits would also need to be adjusted.

There is some empirical evidence suggesting that ethnobiological, ecological, and biomedical information can increase the probability of discovering new drug leads from biological material. Balick (1990) reports that out of 20 plant samples collected in Belize on the basis of ethnobiological data, five showed activity in an in vitro anti-HIV screen conducted by the National Cancer Institute. This compares with only 1 out of 18 Central American plant samples collected at random by Balick that showed activity in the NCI's anti-HIV screen. King and Tempesta (1993) tested extracts of 207 plants collected on the basis of ethnobotanical information. Overall, 42 percent of these plant extracts showed strong activity in three antiviral screening tests. ICBG projects are using ethnobotanical and ecological information as well as more comprehensive (i.e., random) strategies for selecting samples for screening. By the end of 1995, the ICBG projects had screened approximately 2,000 extracts. Of these, 120 have shown significant levels of bioactivity and are of continuing interest, and 25 new drug leads for malaria, cancer, viral diseases, and central nervous system disorders have been isolated and are undergoing further evaluation (Rosenthal 1995). It is worth noting that the ICBG project being conducted in Surinam under the direction of Dr. David Kingston of the Virginia Polytechnic Institute has been designed to compare the success rates of biological samples collected randomly with those collected on the basis of ethnobiological information.

An information-based process for selecting the biological samples to screen is itself a kind of prescreening test. In the case of ethnobotanical information, extracts could even be said to have undergone human trials. Still, higher preliminary screening success rates for ethnobiological or ecologically informed prospecting strategies do not in themselves provide an indication of the superiority of these approaches. For example, if primary screening success rates increase but success rates in dereplication and toxicological evaluation decline in an informed and more narrowly focused prospecting strategy, the net effect could be negative. Higher screening success rates of informed collection strategies must also be balanced against higher research and collection costs and a smaller pool of species that meet the selection criteria. The prospecting organization may also have to accept some limitations on the therapeutic objectives of the program, focusing on those therapeutic areas where traditional knowledge or prior biochemical research have identified potentially effective natural preparations or compounds.

To provide an illustrative example of an ethnobiologically, ecologically, or biomedically informed prospecting strategy, I have made the following changes to the baseline analysis. I have assumed that the prospecting organization is selecting extracts on the basis of expected activity in two therapeutic categories (e.g., anti-inflammatory and anti-infective). I have also assumed that it costs an additional $500 to select and obtain each sample to be tested and that only 5,000 species are expected to meet the selection criteria. Approximately 1,000 extracts could be obtained and screened each year with an expected primary screening success rate of .04. Success rates and testing costs in subsequent R&D phases, as well as expected revenues of a new drug, are assumed to be the same as those incorporated into the baseline analysis. Given these assumptions, the expected before-tax net present value associated with screening the 5,000 extracts that meet the selection criteria would be $6.2 million, compared with a net present value of $7.3 million for screening the 15,000 extracts in the more comprehensive screening program represented by the baseline analysis. However, the average after-tax net present value of each compound in the more focused and informed prospecting strategy is $1,240, compared with $487 for the baseline analysis.

In general, any prospecting strategy must be evaluated in relation to the resources and capabilities of the prospecting organization. A smaller firm with a modest screening capacity and few resources to put at risk may be better served by an informed and focused prospecting strategy. For many large pharmaceutical companies with substantial investments in screening capacity, a random prospecting strategy with high throughput may yield a lower expected present value per extract tested but a higher overall rate of return due to the higher throughput rate and a broader array of screening objectives. This does not mean that large prospecting organizations should ignore ethnobiological, ecological, or biomedical information in developing their screening programs. Rather, large public and private prospecting organizations may do best by combining more comprehensive high throughput screening programs with more selective and informed biochemical prospecting efforts.

Sensitivity Analysis

Assumptions about R&D success rates, potential revenues of a new drug, and the cost of capital can significantly affect estimates of the expected value of screening biological extracts. Prospecting organizations are likely to have significant empirical information on which to base their estimates of the cost of each R&D phase. They are also likely to have developed detailed estimates of the potential market and expected sales of new drugs in the therapeutic areas that are the focus of the prospecting effort. Nevertheless, a significant degree of uncertainty regarding these cost and revenue estimates is still likely to remain. DiMasi and colleagues (1991) and Grabowski and Vernon (1990) found substantial variation in clinical testing costs and revenues of new drug products. In the baseline analysis, an increase (or decrease) of 10 percent in the cost of evaluating a compound in each postscreening R&D phase reduces (increases) the before-tax *ENPV* by almost $7.3 million. An increase (decrease) of 10 percent in expected revenues of each new drug increases (decreases) the *ENPV* of the baseline analysis by approximately $11 million.

Changes in the cost of capital or discount rate have perhaps the most significant effect on the expected value of the prospecting effort simply because significant R&D expenditures must be made many years in advance of potential revenues. If the discount rate in the baseline analysis is increased from 8.5 to 9 percent, the *ENPV* of the proposed screening program becomes negative. Conversely, if the discount rate in the baseline analysis is reduced from 8.5 to 8 percent, the *ENPV* of the prospecting effort increases from $7 million to $18 million.

One scenario worth examining involves a simultaneous increase in the discount rate and expected revenues. Such a situation could be generated from an aging population that is drawing down its savings. If the discount rate is increased to 9 percent and expected new drug revenues are increased by 10 percent, the net effect on the baseline analysis is a decrease of approximately $150,000 relative to the *ENPV* of the baseline analysis.

The remaining set of critical parameters in the model are the expected success rates of each R&D phase. In general, a reduction in the success rate of any phase will reduce the expected value of the screening program. However, changes in the expected success rates of later R&D phases have a proportionately greater impact on the expected value of the program. In the baseline analysis, if the anticipated primary screening success rate is reduced by 20 percent—from .005 to .004—the pretax *ENPV* of the prospecting effort is reduced from $7.3 million to $2.9 million. But, if the conditional success rate of preclinical testing is reduced by 20 percent—from .4 to .32—the expected net present value of the prospecting opportunity becomes negative.

This illustrates that debates over the number of compounds which must be tested to develop one new drug are meaningless. In both of these cases, approximately 140,000 biological extracts would have to be tested to identify a novel compound that will eventually lead to a new drug in any given therapeutic category. The difference in the expected value of screening each extract in these two cases is due to differences in how quickly unsuccessful new drug leads are identified and dropped from further testing. In fact, many natural product screening programs are consciously designed to have low hit rates in preliminary and even secondary screening so that the very substantial expenditures of subsequent R&D phases are lavished on only the most promising new leads. The critical issue is to set the sensitivity of the screening program at the point where the costs of false positives are approximately equal to the foregone benefits of false negatives.

It seems logical to assume that discovery of one or more novel chemical compounds with promise in a particular therapeutic area will reduce the probability of discovering other novel chemical compounds in that therapeutic area as screening continues. The empirical question is how significant this effect will be on the success rate of the dereplication phase. This issue was discussed above in formulating Equation 2.13, where r was loosely defined as the degree of chemical correlation between the extracts being tested. If we increase r in the baseline analysis from 0 to 0.10, the pretax *ENPV* of the prospecting effort declines from \$7.3 to \$2.3 million. Moreover, the declining success rate of the dereplication phase causes a decline in the value of screening each additional extract. Screening the first extract has an *ENPV* of \$487, while the ENPV of screening the last of the 15,000 extracts is negative. The implications of a declining dereplication phase success rate with regard to the optimal number of extracts to screen is discussed more fully later in this chapter. The results of the sensitivity analyses outlined above are summarized in Table 2.3.

Up to this point, I have discussed the critical parameters in the model in terms of single value estimates. However, it is more realistic and more useful to characterize assumptions about the value of these parameters in terms of a probability distribution of possible values. The single value estimates previously utilized in the analysis can be understood as the means of these distributions. For parameter estimates based upon a significant body of empirical data, the probability distribution would be tightly grouped around the mean. Conversely, where very little empirical information is available, the probability distribution of possible values for success rates, R&D phase costs, or new drug revenues would be more dispersed. Given

TABLE 2.3. Summary of Sensitivity Analysis

	Baseline	Increased R&D Costs	Increased Revenues	Increased Disc. Rate	Decreased Disc. Rate	Low Primary Screening Success Rate	Low Preclinical Success Rate	High Chemical Correlation
Modified Parameters:								
Extracts Tested	15,000	15,000	15,000	15,000	15,000	15,000	15,000	15,000
Chem. Correlation	0.0	0.0	0.0	0.0	0.0	0.0	0.0	0.1
Real Discount Rate	8.50%	8.50%	8.50%	9.00%	8.00%	8.50%	8.50%	8.50%
Prim. Screen Success Rate	0.005	0.005	0.005	0.005	0.005	0.004	0.005	0.005
Preclin. Success Rate	0.40	0.40	0.40	0.40	0.40	0.40	0.32	0.40
R&D Cost Multiplier	1.00	1.10	1.00	1.00	1.00	1.00	1.00	1.00
New Drug Revenue Multiplier	1.00	1.00	1.10	1.00	1.00	1.00	1.00	1.00
Results:								
Expected NPV – Total	$7,300,473	$12,434	$18,076,205	($2,453,678)	$18,462,339	$2,930,767	($1,508,825)	$2,260,378
Expected NPV – First Extract	$487	$1	$1,205	($164)	$1,231	$195	($101)	$487
Expected NPV – Last Extract	$487	$1	$1,205	($164)	$1,231	$195	($101)	($1)
Expected NPV – Avg. per Extract	$487	$1	$1,205	($164)	$1,231	$195	($101)	$151

a plausible set of probability distributions, simulation models can be used to provide an improved understanding of the variability of outcomes from the prospecting effort.

Figure 2.5 summarizes the results of a Monte Carlo simulation where the parameter values used in the baseline analysis are used as the means of a set of probability distributions for these parameters. More detailed data on the assumptions and results of the simulation are provided in Appendix A. One important result of the simulation is that the median net present value is negative after 200 iterations (which could be thought of as 200 prospecting projects). Given probability distributions for R&D phase costs, success rates, new drug revenues, and the cost of capital as defined in the simulation, most biochemical prospecting projects would not yield a return equal to what could be obtained from alternative investments. How-

FIGURE 2.5. Distribution of Returns from Monte Carlo Simulation of Prospecting Opportunity

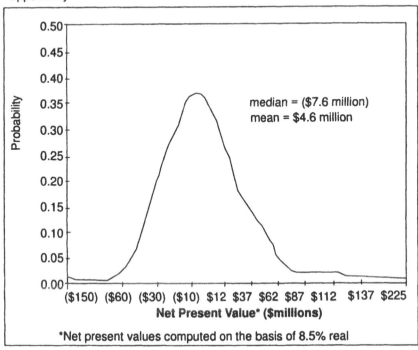

median = ($7.6 million)
mean = $4.6 million

*Net present values computed on the basis of 8.5% real

ever, a few of the iterations (projects) in the analysis generate very high returns, which causes the mean net present value of the simulation to be positive. Similar results were obtained by Grabowski and Vernon (1990) in their empirical analysis of the returns of 100 new pharmaceutical products. It is the possibility of discovering a major new drug that makes pharmaceutical research profitable.

Estimating the Expected Value of Information

In the baseline analysis, obtaining access to a supply of unscreened biological extracts has a positive expected net present value. However, as demonstrated by the sensitivity and simulation analyses, proceeding with a biochemical screening program is a risky investment. Any number of estimates in the baseline analysis could turn out to be overly optimistic and result in the prospecting effort yielding negative net present values. By extending the decision theoretic framework already presented, it is possible to estimate the expected value of obtaining exact knowledge about the values of critical parameters in the analysis. In the terminology of decision analysis, this is referred to as the expected value of perfect information ($EVPI$). Although perfect information is rarely, if ever, available in the real world, estimating the $EVPI$ lays the groundwork for evaluating the expected value of imperfect information, which in turn can be used to estimate how many extracts to screen and when to terminate an ongoing screening program. To illustrate the potential benefits of obtaining new information, I will focus on the success rate assumed for preliminary screening tests.

A convenient way of summarizing the expectation and level of certainty of the prospecting organization with regard to the success rate of the primary screening phase is through the use of a beta distribution. The parameters α and β, which define a beta distribution, can be thought of as the number of successes and failures in a screening test with sample size $(\alpha + \beta)$, mean $\alpha/(\alpha + \beta)$, and variance $\beta/(\alpha + \beta)^2(\alpha + \beta + 1)$. If the prospecting organization has a high degree of confidence regarding its judgment of the primary screening success rate, this would be reflected by selecting relatively large values for α and β. Smaller values of α and β would indicate a lower level of certainty regarding the expected success rate.

For example, let's assume the prospecting organization has some information on the primary screening success rate of a previous biochemical prospecting effort that had a similar therapeutic objective. But this previous prospecting effort involved different criteria for selecting biological samples and a different type of primary screening test. The primary screening success rate for this previous prospecting effort was .01, but for the above reasons, the prospecting organization is not particularly confident that a new prospecting opportunity will have a similar primary success rate. The organization believes there is a reasonable chance that the rate could be as high as .025 or as low as .001, but the mean is probably closer to .01. These judgmental assessments might be represented by a beta distribution with parameters $\alpha = 1$, $\beta = 99$.

Alternatively, a prospecting organization may have reviewed the results of numerous other prospecting efforts and be quite confident that the primary screening success rate for its new screening program will turn out to be very close to .01. In this case, the prospecting organization might use a beta distribution with $\alpha = 10$, $\beta = 990$ to represent its expectations and level of certainty regarding the primary screening success rate.

Given values of α and β that reflect the expected value of the primary screening success rate and the level of certainty in that estimate, the probability of realizing an average success rate of greater than a and less than b, can be computed from the beta density function as follows:

$$p(s_1) \subset [a,b] = \frac{\Gamma(\alpha+\beta)}{\Gamma(\alpha)\Gamma(\beta)} \int_a^b s_1^{\alpha-1} (1-s_1)^{\beta-1} ds_1 \qquad (2.15)$$

where a and b lie in the closed interval $[0,1]$, s_1 is the average primary screen success rate for each screening test, and the first term in the equation is a scaling factor where

$$\Gamma(X) = \int_0^\infty y^{x-1} e^{-y} dy \qquad (2.15a)$$

Using this equation and the estimated costs and expected success rates of subsequent R&D phases, it is possible to estimate the expected value of obtaining perfect information about the success rate of the primary screening phase. Let $ENPV^*|s_1$ be the expected net present value *of the best course of action,* given an average success rate of s_I in primary screening for each therapeutic indicator. The expected net present value of the prospecting opportunity, given perfect information about the primary screening success rate, can then be computed as follows:

$$ENPV|PI(s_1) = \frac{\Gamma(\alpha+\beta)}{\Gamma(\alpha)\Gamma(\beta)} \int_0^1 s_1^{\alpha-1}(1-s_1)^{\beta-1} \, ENPV^*|s_1 ds_1 \quad (2.16)$$

The expected value of perfect information about the success rate in the primary screening phase is, therefore, the difference between *ENPV|PI(s_I)* and the *ENPV* of the best course of action based upon prior information.

The Expected Value of Sample Information

The calculation of *EVPI* places an upper bound on the costs that should be accepted to obtain imperfect or sample information. If the *ENPV* of the proposed prospecting opportunities were positive, the prospecting organization would proceed and the question would become how to monitor and respond to preliminary results of the program. This issue is addressed at the end of this section. However, when the *ENPV* of screening an extract is negative, there is an expected cost for obtaining additional information about screening success rates, which must be compared with the expected value of that information.

Conceptually, the process of computing the expected value of sample information *(EVSI)* is quite similar to that described above for *EVPI*. If the prospecting organization decides to screen a sample of x extracts, there are $x + 1$ different possible results from the sample data. Given the organization's prior judgment about the primary screening success rate (again represented by a beta distribution), the expected frequency of each potential sample result can be approximated from the beta density function:

$$p(a) \cong \frac{\Gamma(\alpha+\beta)}{\Gamma(\alpha-1)\Gamma(\beta-1)} \int_{(a-.5) \div x}^{(a+.5) \div x} s_1^{\alpha-1}(1-s_1)^{\beta-1} \, ds_1 \quad (2.17)$$

where a is the number of positive test results in the sample, x is the number of compounds tested, and α, β are the parameters of the beta distribution that represents the prior judgments about the success rate in each primary screening test. (For $a = 0$, the lower limit of the integral should be set at 0 and for $a = x$, the upper limit at 1).

The actual primary screening success rate of the sample will provide information with which to update the prospecting organization's prior judgment regarding the primary screening success rate. A convenient way of doing this is to pool the data resulting from the sample with the beta distribution that represents the prior judgment of the success rate. The resulting distribution is referred to as the posterior probability distribution and is a weighted combination of prior information and the results of the sample. The mean of the posterior distribution can be calculated as shown below:

$$\widetilde{s}_1 = \frac{(\alpha + a)}{(\alpha + \beta + x)} \tag{2.18}$$

For a prospecting opportunity with a negative prior estimate of *ENPV*, the *EVSI(s_1)* is simply the *ENPV* of the prospecting endeavor after incorporating the expected results of the sample. Equation 2.19 below summarizes this calculation:

$$EVSI(s_1) = \sum_{a=0}^{x} p(a)(ENPV^* | \widetilde{s}_1) \tag{2.19}$$

Even though *EVSI(s_1)* might be positive, it may still be less than the expected cost of screening a sample of x extracts. The critical value is, therefore, the expected value of sample information net of sampling costs (*NEVSI*). Given a prior expectation of a negative net present value of proceeding with a prospecting opportunity, the *NEVSI* for the primary screening success rate can be calculated as follows:

$$NEVSI(s_1) = EVSI(s_1) - \sum_{i=1}^{x} [\min (c_0 + c_1), |ENPV_i|] \tag{2.20}$$

where c_0 and c_1 are the costs of obtaining and screening each extract respectively, N is the potential number of extracts that could be obtained from the prospecting opportunity, and $|ENPV_i|$ is the ex ante absolute expected value of screening the ith extract.

Determining the Optimum Number of Samples to Screen

The value of x in Equation 2.20 that yields the maximum value of $NEVSI(s_l)$ would be the optimum sample size (x^*) for gathering additional information on the value of s_l. If the prospecting organization is quite confident about its prior estimate of s_l, then $EVSI(s_l)$ will be relatively low for all sample sizes and the optimal sample size might be zero (i.e., $NEVSI(s_l) < 0$ for all $x > 0$). However, if the prospecting organization has very little prior information about s_l (i.e., the prior probability distribution of s_l has a relatively large variance) then $EVSI(s_l)$ and x^* will be greater, all other things being equal.

A spreadsheet or simple computer program can be used to calculate approximate values for $EVSI(s_l)$, $NEVSI(s_l)$, and x^*. For a prospecting opportunity where s_l is represented by a beta distribution with $\alpha = .1$, $\beta = 99.9$, and all other parameters are the same as the baseline analysis, the $ENPV$ of screening all 15,000 extracts is negative. Faced with a choice of procuring access to all 15,000 samples or pursuing some other equally risky investment with a real rate of return equal to 8.5 percent, the prospecting organization would choose the latter. However, in this situation there is a positive value associated with gathering sample information about the primary screening success rate. As shown in Figure 2.6, the optimum sample size for this prospecting opportunity outlined above is approximately 600 extracts, and the expected value of this sample information net of screening costs is approximately $800,000. For sample sizes greater than 600, the expected benefit of gaining increased statistical certainty about the primary screening success rate begins to be more than offset by the expected cost of screening additional extracts.

Sample information about success rates and phase costs is continually being generated as the prospecting effort proceeds. Utilizing the methodology outlined above for incorporating both prior judgments (or prior data) and new sample information into a posterior distribution, the prospecting organization could use the preliminary results of the program to periodically revise its estimates of the expected value of screening additional extracts. If the $ENPV$ of continuing to test biological extracts becomes negative, the pros-

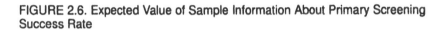

FIGURE 2.6. Expected Value of Sample Information About Primary Screening Success Rate

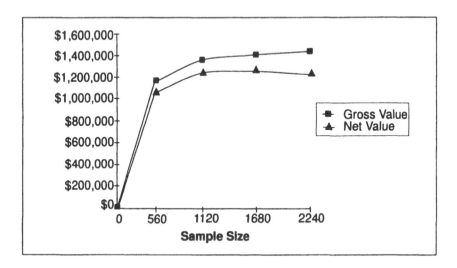

pecting organization should estimate the expected value of obtaining additional information (*NEVSI*) before terminating the screening program. Only if the *NEVSI* that could be derived from continued screening becomes negative should the screening program be terminated.

Considerations about the optimum number of extracts to screen and when to terminate or redirect an ongoing screening program also arise due to an expectation of a declining success rate in the dereplication phase and the increasing possibility that more than one new drug might be discovered for a given therapeutic objective. These considerations can be incorporated into the prospecting organization's decisions analysis in the form of an optimization problem with respect to the number of extracts to screen, as shown in Equation 2.21 below:

$$\max_{N} enpv = \sum_{k=1}^{N} \left[pvb \prod_{i=1}^{n} (s_i)(1 - \prod_{i=1}^{n} s_i)^k - \sum_{j=1}^{n} pvc \prod_{i=1}^{j-1} (s_i) \right] \qquad (2.21)$$

where *pvb* is the present value of benefits of a new drug net of marketing and manufacturing costs, *N* is the number of extracts to screen, n is the number of phases in the R&D process, pvc_j is the present value cost of testing a compound or extract in phase j, and the success rate in the dereplication phase incorporates the relationship defined in Equation 2.13.

A variation of the optimization problem defined above can be used to determine when to stop screening new extracts. In this case, the prospecting organization must take into account the actual trend in dereplication phase success rates and the progress of extracts or isolated compounds through the R&D process. Obviously, the decision to continue screening depends on whether the expected net benefits of doing so are positive, which can be determined from the following equation:

$$enpv = \left[pvb \prod_{i=1}^{n} (s_i)(1 - \sum_{k=1}^{p} \prod_{j=c_k}^{n} s_j) - \sum_{j=1}^{n} pvc_j \prod_{i=1}^{j-1} (s_i) \right] \quad (2.22)$$

where p is the number of previously screened extracts that have not yet failed any phase of the R&D process, c_k is the next phase in which compound k must be tested, and the success rate in the dereplication phase is again defined by Equation 2.13.

The Option Value of Pharmaceutical R&D

The basic model developed thus far includes only two outcomes—success and failure—for each screening test or trial. However, at any stage of the R&D process, with the possible exception of regulatory review of a new drug application, outcomes can take on a continuous range of values. A compound that showed highly positive test results in preclinical trials would be expected to have a greater possibility of success in clinical trials than a compound that resulted in significant but not exceptional test results. A more detailed and informative model would therefore include a greater number, or even a continuous distribution, of test results for each phase of the R&D process.

For example, the potential results of each R&D phase could be categorized as highly positive (++), positive but not highly positive (+), and insignificant or negative (−). In addition, the expected probabilities associated with each of these results in any phase, except the first, are contingent on test results from the previous phase. Figure 2.7 depicts a partial decision tree for this expanded model. For ease of presentation, the tree has been folded back to the end of the second phase of the R&D process. The expected net present value of a compound that has highly positive test results in Phase II is denoted by $enpv_2|(2++)$. Similarly, the expected value of a compound that has shown positive but not highly positive test results in Phase II is denoted by $enpv_2|(2+)$.

There are several advantages to a model with more detailed specification of the possible results of each R&D phase. First, it forces the prospecting organization to think more systematically about the correlation between test results of compounds in consecutive phases. This set of relationships is critical to determining the threshold test values above which compounds are deemed worthy of further R&D expenditures. In addition, a more detailed specification enables the prospecting organization to estimate with greater accuracy the expected value of a compound at any stage of the R&D process. Finally, incorporating greater detail into the model permits the prospecting organization to benefit more fully from the information contained in the results of the ongoing prospecting effort.

Another useful aspect of specifying a model with a range of test results in each R&D phase is that it serves to highlight the relationship between the expected value of a compound after completion of a particular R&D phase and the compound's test results in that phase, as shown in Figure 2.8. Performing a particular test or trial is like purchasing a call option. If the results of the test are below some critical threshold, the expected value of pursuing subsequent R&D on the compound will be less than zero and the option of doing so will go unexercised. However, as test results rise above that critical threshold, the value of exercising the option to proceed with further R&D on that compound continues to increase, although not necessarily in a linear fashion. This relationship is illustrated in Figure 2.8.

The analogy to an option on a financial security can be pressed a bit further by considering a biological extract that has been tested in primary screening assays. In this situation, the prospecting organization has the option to subject the extract to secondary screening tests. The purchase price of this option is the cost of secondary screening. The expected value of the option will depend on both the

FIGURE 2.7. Partial Decision Tree for More Complex Model

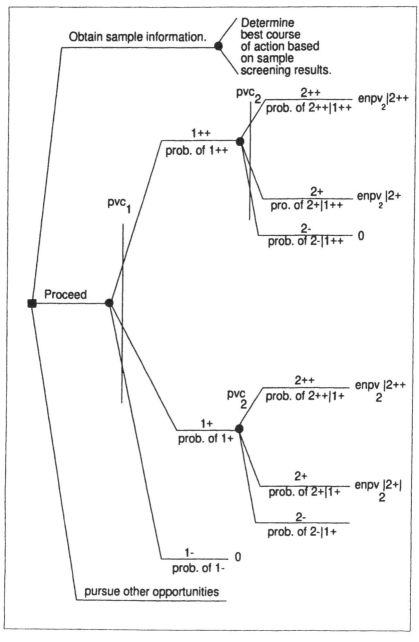

FIGURE 2.8. Expected Value of a Compound as a Function of Test Results in Current Phase

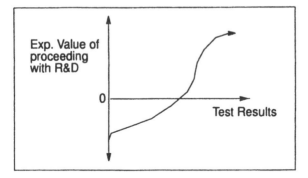

critical threshold above which secondary screening results are deemed to be positive and the potential variance of secondary screening results, given the extract's primary screening test results. If the prospecting organization purchases the option (i.e., if it proceeds with secondary screening), it should only exercise the option (i.e., continue with subsequent R&D) if the secondary screening test results exceed the "exercise value," or critical threshold above which results are deemed to be positive.

For a proposed prospecting opportunity where the underlying asset is a large supply of biological samples, the application of standard option pricing models is complicated by the potential for chemical and therapeutic redundancy discussed earlier in this chapter. Discovery of one or more valuable new chemicals may reduce the value of screening additional extracts. This is analogous to a situation where the holder of financial options would significantly affect the market price of the underlying assets by the exercise of those options. These complications notwithstanding, the potential loss involved in screening a biological extract or compound is limited to the cost of performing the screening test, but the potential gain is limited only by the potential revenues or social benefits that would result from discovery of one or more new drugs. Since the range of potential benefits associated with positive results is much greater than the potential cost of negative test results, a high variance in expected test results is a positive asset. The more diverse the supply of extracts is, the greater the expected variance in screening test results and the greater the expected value of proceeding with the prospecting opportunity. This would imply that a prospecting organization can increase the expected return from biochemical prospecting activities by screening extracts from widely divergent taxa, biogeographic regions, life stages, ecological niches, etc.

POTENTIAL APPLICATIONS AND EXTENSIONS OF THE MODEL

Before highlighting potential applications of the model, I would first like to offer a few notes of caution regarding the interpretation of the model and some of the sample calculations. Although I utilized recent empirical data and information provided by pharmaceutical researchers to develop the parameters in the baseline analysis, the results should not be interpreted as an estimate of the value of preserving a species until it can be screened for pharmaceutical potential. To evaluate properly the pharmaceutical value of preserving a species or an ecosystem, it would be necessary to consider a comprehensive set of therapeutic targets, to develop an improved understanding of the degree of chemical redundancy across species and taxonomic groups, and to consider the effects of changes in technology and demand for pharmaceutical products over time. The results of the model also should not be interpreted as providing an indication of the market value of biological extracts. Since the models presented in this chapter only consider the demand for biological extracts, the results only provide an estimate of the upper limit of potential market value. Supply-side considerations and the value of preserving species and ecosystems for biochemical prospecting are considered in subsequent chapters.

The primary intention of this chapter was to demonstrate how a prospecting organization could use the basic model—together with its own estimates of success rates, R&D costs, and potential revenues—to evaluate ongoing or proposed biochemical prospecting projects. In the baseline analysis, I have used a risk-adjusted discount rate as a proxy for other investment opportunities. In doing so, I have implicitly assumed that these other investment opportunities have risk characteristics that are similar to the proposed biochemical prospecting project. In some cases, a more detailed analysis that explicitly compares the potential range of competing R&D investment options may be more appropriate. The option of gathering additional information before committing to a major program should also be included in the analysis.

Any direct comparison of R&D options should begin with an estimation of the potential range of outcomes, their probability of occurrence, and their correlation with other investments of the prospecting organization. This information, together with a risk-free discount rate and a utility function that reflects the prospecting organization's risk preferences, could then be used to determine if the prospecting effort is preferred to other investment opportunities (Smith and Nau 1992).

Another important application of the basic model is as a tool for monitoring and evaluating ongoing biochemical screening programs. Ongoing programs generate a wealth of information about preliminary screening success rates, screening costs, dereplication and chemical redundancy, and the prospects of new leads gaining regulatory approval as new drugs. All of this information can be incorporated into the model to reevaluate, and if necessary revise, the prospecting effort. Lower than expected screening success rates could require fine tuning of the success criteria or the application of different bioassays. Increasing rates of chemical redundancy in the extracts that test positively in preliminary screens could indicate the need to obtain a greater diversity of biological samples. Or, under the best of circumstances, discovery of several promising leads in one therapeutic category could justify the substitution of other therapeutic targets in the ongoing screening program.

The basic model outlined in this chapter can also be extended in a number of ways to address other management decisions faced by organizations involved in pharmaceutical R&D. For example, a model with a range of potential outcomes for preliminary screening results could be used to evaluate the implicit tradeoff between the costs of false positives and false negatives involved in setting success criteria for preliminary screening. A less stringent set of criteria for selecting compounds that should proceed to subsequent R&D phases would reduce the probability that valuable compounds would go unrecognized but would also increase R&D costs. A more stringent success criteria reduces R&D costs but also increases the probability that new drug leads will be eliminated from further consideration before their value can be recognized. The underlying assumptions involved in establishing a given success criteria can be quantified and subjected to more systematic evaluation with the aid of the model.

In many natural product screening programs, primary screening of extracts can now be done quite rapidly. However, a critical bottleneck can occur due to the additional time and more specialized skills involved in chemical isolation, dereplication, and modification of compounds. By incorporating a queuing theory application into the general model, it would be possible to estimate the optimal rate at which to procure and screen biological extracts, given certain assumptions about the primary screening success rate and knowledge of the resources available for subsequent R&D phases. In addition, if data were available on how various combinations of personnel and capital equipment affect productivity and success rates at various stages of the R&D process, this information could be integrated into the model to allow for more efficient decisions regarding the scale and configuration of the R&D program.

Although I have focused on pharmaceutical natural product research in this chapter, the models and analytic techniques presented can easily be applied to evaluate other natural product R&D programs or to evaluate other forms of pharmaceutical R&D. By adjusting the number of phases, the success rates (or probability distributions over outcomes), the costs and duration of each phase, and the expected revenues from each new product, the basic model can be used to assess the value of biological material as a source of new agrochemicals, industrial feedstocks, fragrances, and flavors, as well as a source of genetic material for agricultural breeding programs.

Chapter 3

Host Country Options for Conservation and Sustainable Development

INTRODUCTION

Population growth, agricultural expansion, and industrial development are causing degradation of large areas of species-rich habitat throughout the world (FAO 1990; Reid 1992). Although natural ecosystems often provide significant benefits, such as watershed protection, carbon sequestration, and ecotourist revenues, the magnitude, timing, and distribution of these benefits generally have not provided central governments or local populations with sufficient economic incentives to preserve primal forests, wetlands, coral reefs, and other biologically diverse ecosystems. The possibility of discovering valuable biochemical compounds is an additional justification for preserving natural ecosystems, and for some biologically rich habitats, the potential benefits of biochemical prospecting could tip the balance in favor of conservation. To evaluate how biochemical prospecting could or should affect land-use decisions and development strategies, it is necessary to define the benefits of potential prospecting activities, to understand how they will be distributed among affected parties, and to incorporate this information into a comprehensive framework for economic decision making.

A country can be reactive or proactive in the development of its biological resources. In responding to specific biochemical prospecting proposals, evaluating their merits, and attempting to amend the proposed terms to increase expected benefits, the host government is operating in a reactive mode. A proactive management approach would involve some combination of ecological research, habitat protection, international marketing efforts, and development of the country's own biochemical research and development capabilities. In reality, a biologically rich country is likely to be simultaneously involved in both reactive and proactive efforts to develop its biological resources.

The first section of this chapter presents a general analytical framework for economic evaluation of a proposed biochemical prospecting effort.[1] The second section presents an analytical framework for incorporating the potential benefits of biochemical prospecting into the host country's land-use plans. The final section discusses strategies for developing, marketing, and distributing the benefits of the host country's biochemical resources.

EVALUATING A PROPOSED BIOCHEMICAL PROSPECTING OPPORTUNITY

The first step in evaluating any investment opportunity is to determine what alternative investments would be precluded by proceeding with the opportunity being investigated. In the case of a proposed biochemical prospecting program, the critical issue is where the prospecting would occur and what potential uses of those areas, if any, would have to be altered or postponed to conduct the prospecting effort. If the contract would provide the prospecting organization, or its agent(s), with access to a well-defined geographic area and prohibit further development in that area for a specified period of time, the foregone net benefits of land-use conversion (i.e., opportunity costs) are easily defined. However, in many cases the proposed contract may not occur in a predefined location. For example, the contract may only require the host country, or a third-party collector, to deliver a predetermined list of biological samples or extracts. However, even in this case, failure to protect certain natural areas could reduce the income generated from the prospecting effort if habitat conversion or encroachment prevented the host country from obtaining initial or subsequent samples of some species.

Perhaps the simplest situation to analyze is where the proposed prospecting location is a national park or biological reserve that is already benefiting from effective protection and management. In this case, the prospecting contract is not precluding any alternative uses of the site. A similar situation may arise even if the prospecting location is not a legally protected area but is sufficiently remote from population centers and transportation links to preclude most alternate uses. Of course, if there are no competing land-uses, the host country still has the option of refusing the prospecting opportunity and leaving the prospecting location(s) undisturbed. This might be the preferred alternative if the proposed contract would in some way limit the host country's future uses of the site or the biological resources found there. With no competing land-uses, the decision about whether to proceed with the prospecting contract should therefore be represented by a decision tree with two branches, as shown in Figure 3.1.

An additional branch should be added to the decision tree if the proposed prospecting location is also a valuable site for incompatible agricultural, forestry, or mining activities. In this case, the expected benefits of the prospecting contract must be compared with the foregone net benefits of leaving the site undisturbed or converting the site to another land-use, as shown in Figure 3.2.

In many cases, alternative uses of the prospecting location cannot be neatly defined as compatible or incompatible, but lie along a more or less continuous scale of compatibility. Clear-cutting all, or a significant portion, of a primary forest would reduce the number of species from which samples could be collected. But a selective logging program that harvested only a small number of species might have relatively little impact on the absolute number of biological samples that could be collected from the site (A. D. Johns 1992; R. J. Johns 1992). Similarly, conversion of a natural area into

FIGURE 3.1. Decision Tree with No Competing Land-Uses

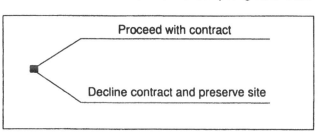

FIGURE 3.2. Decision Tree with Site Conversion Alternative

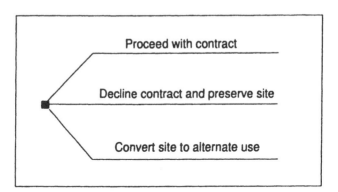

a combination of mixed-use agriculture and agroforestry interspersed with remnants of natural vegetation might reduce local biodiversity but still preserve a substantial portion of it (Brown and Brown 1992; Schelhas 1994). If the proposed prospecting contract leaves the host country free to decide what combination and magnitude of other economic activities to permit at the prospecting locations, then the host country must consider what mix of biochemical prospecting and other land-uses will yield the maximum expected utility.

If the prospecting contract does not specify a particular prospecting location but only requires delivery of a predetermined list of distinct biological samples or extracts, the host country must determine where these organisms can be found and what, if any, economic activities may endanger them during the course of the contract. The risks that various land-uses or economic activities might pose to particular species, together with the expected income that would be lost due to an inability to obtain samples from any of the species on the list, would have to be compared with the costs of habitat preservation in the relevant parts of the country. Forecasting what type and how much development would otherwise occur at the potential prospecting locations. What risks that development would pose to the species of interest, and what economic surpluses would be foregone due to any prohibitions against certain economic activities would be a difficult task even for countries with well-developed biological and economic research programs. In practice, the host country might focus its attention on identifying what species of interest to the prospecting organization have relatively small population sizes and/or geographic ranges and then evaluate the costs and benefits of strategies for protecting these populations.

Direct Benefits and Costs

The direct benefits of a proposed prospecting contract are likely to include a combination of guaranteed and contingent compensation. Guaranteed compensation would include all forms of payment, training, or technology transfer that are not dependent on the success of the prospecting effort. A common feature of many recent prospecting arrangements is a fixed payment for the delivery of a specified supply of biological samples. Although the payment is contingent on the ability of the host country, or its agents, to obtain and deliver the desired samples, the events that could affect the host country's compensation are largely within its control. This is not the case with contingent compensation arrangements such as royalties or profit-sharing agreements. Royalties, which are usually defined as a percentage of gross revenues, are contingent on both the number of successful products developed from the prospecting effort and the revenues ultimately derived from each product. Under a profit-sharing arrangement, both the host country's compensation and the net benefits received by the prospecting organization are contingent not only on the number of successful products and the revenues generated by each but also on the costs associated with research, development, marketing, and production.

If the host country is risk neutral, the direct net benefits of a prospecting contract involving guaranteed compensation and prospective royalties can be summarized as follows. Let G_t be any guaranteed payments to be made by the prospecting firm in year t, let TT_t be the value of technology transfer and technical assistance provided in year t, let p be the amount paid by the prospecting organization upon receipt of each extract or biological sample, let EGR_t be the expected gross revenues in year t derived from new drugs developed from the prospecting effort, let π be the percentage of gross revenues from new drugs that will be paid to the host country, let c be the average cost of collecting and preparing each biological sample for delivery to the prospecting organization, and let C_t be the additional costs in year t for protection and management of the prospecting location(s). In addition, let D be the period during which extracts or samples will be delivered to the prospecting organization, let x_t be the number of extracts collected in year t, let Y be the expected time before marketing of a new drug, let T be the expected commercial life of a new drug, and let δ be the risk-neutral discount rate for the host country. The expected present value of the direct benefits of the prospecting contract are therefore:

$$DNB = \sum_{t=1}^{D} [G_t + TT_t + (p - c) x_t - C_t](1+\delta)^{-t} + \pi \sum_{t=Y}^{Y+T} EGR_t(1+\delta)^{-t}$$

(3.1)

As described in the preceding chapter, expected gross revenues, EGR_t, will depend on the specific objectives of the prospecting program as well as the prospecting strategies, screening technologies, and level of effort employed by the prospecting organization. If the host country has some knowledge of the prospecting organization's research objectives and methodologies and has access to data on screening technologies and new drug revenues, Equations 2.4 and 2.5 can be used to calculate expected gross revenues. Substituting into Equation 3.1 yields

$$DNB = \sum_{t=1}^{D} [G_t + TT_t + (p - c) x_t - C_t](1+\delta)^{-t} + \pi MN \prod_{i=1}^{n} s_i \sum_{t=Y}^{Y+T} R_t(1+\delta)^{-t}$$

(3.2)

where N is the total number of biological samples that will be collected and screened as part of the contract, M is the number of different product categories that are being screened for, s_i is the contingent probability of an extract or isolated compound advancing through stage i of the R&D program, and R_t is the revenue generated in year t by the average new product in the product categories that are the focus of the prospecting effort.

The value of any technology transfer and technical assistance included in the proposed contract should generally be estimated in terms of the avoided costs of obtaining similar equipment, training, or technology licenses from other sources. However, there may be no alternative source of supply for proprietary technology or no other means of obtaining access to the results of research on the extracts obtained through the contract. In this case, the host country must estimate the incremental net revenues or public benefits that can expected from access to this proprietary technology or information. One way of approaching this problem is to utilize the models presented in the previous chapter to quantify the expected net present value of the host country's biochemical R&D programs with and without the proprietary information or technology.

The economic alternatives for the prospecting location(s) may include combinations of biochemical prospecting activities and ecologically disruptive land-uses. Calculation of the direct benefits of these mixed-use alternatives must include both the expected net revenues from partial conversion of the natural ecosystem at the site and the expected direct benefits from biochemical prospecting, given the effects of these other land-uses on the biodiversity of the area. It is also essential to incorporate into the decision analysis the fact that some land-use choices will preclude future options. In the extreme case, complete conversion of the prospecting locations would not only preclude the proposed prospecting contract but would also prevent significant prospecting efforts at these sites in the foreseeable future. The dynamic effects of current land-use choices are discussed in more detail later in this chapter.

For a prospecting contract that does not specify particular prospecting locations but instead requires delivery of a list of biological samples, calculation of expected direct net benefits could still follow the methodology summarized in Equation 3.2. In this case, only the costs of protecting the habitats of relatively rare or particularly fragile species on the list would be incorporated into the analysis. It is these critical habitats that would also be analyzed with regard to the potential benefits of alternative, incompatible land-uses.

Environmental Services and Compatible Land-Use Benefits

In addition to the direct benefits and costs associated with biochemical prospecting and alternative land-uses, there are a number of indirect costs and benefits that should be incorporated into the analysis if one or more of the options in the decision analysis involves land-use conversion. These include the environmental benefits associated with preservation of all or some of the prospecting location(s) and the expected revenues from other relatively compatible economic activities (e.g., extractive reserves, ecotourism).[2]

Natural ecosystems often provide numerous goods and services that can be sustainably managed for household consumption or small-scale commercial production. Depending on both the socio-economic characteristics of the human community and the biophysical attributes of the ecosystem, these goods and services might include food, fuel, building materials, medicines, a regular supply of fresh water, and a source of spiritual inspiration. To appropriately account for these additional benefits of the natural ecosystem, it is essential to determine whether the alternative land-uses that are being compared with the prospecting opportunity can provide some of these same services. Complete conversion of a forested ecosystem into cattle pasture would eliminate most, if not all, of the other extractive uses and environmental amenities. However, if the potential alternative uses of the site are mixed-use agriculture and agroforestry activities interspersed with remnants of the natural ecosystem, the converted landscape may still provide many of the benefits associated with complete preservation (Schelhas 1994; Brown and Brown 1992; Saunders, Hobbs, and Margules 1991). It is therefore important to estimate the benefits of small-scale extraction, recreation, and environmental services that would be realized under all land-use options being considered in the decision analysis.

As centers of high species diversity, desirable prospecting locations may also be potential ecotourist destinations. With some limitations on the number of visitors and the type of support services provided, ecotourist activities can comfortably coexist with most biochemical prospecting programs. The potential for ecotourism revenues may be reduced, but not necessarily eliminated, by land-use options that involve partial conversion of the natural habitat at the prospecting locations. As with small-scale extraction and environmental services, potential ecotourist revenues should be estimated for each prospecting and land-use alternative being considered.

Existence Value

Many people place a positive value on the preservation of a species or natural ecosystem, even if they believe these elements of nature will never provide any commercial, material, or direct aesthetic benefits. These individuals value the mere existence of the relevant species or ecosystem. Unfortunately, like many other benefits of environmental conservation, there is no fully functional market that provides an indication of the magnitude of existence value. Although political involvement with or financial contributions to environmental causes can provide some indication of the value that individuals place on environmental protection, it is difficult to disentangle existence values from other direct and indirect benefits associated with environmental preservation. Direct surveys, known as contingent valuation (CV) models, have often been used to estimate the benefits of preserving wilderness areas or individual species. However, there is continuing debate about the accuracy of these survey techniques in estimating existence values (Hausman 1993).

Although difficult to measure, ethical considerations and existence values should, at a minimum, cause an examination of all feasible land-use options. In many cases, leaving remnants of natural habitat, buffer zones, and corridors to larger protected areas can preserve a significant portion of a region's biodiversity while still providing significant land area for other economic activities (Saunders, Hobbs, and Margules 1991; Brown and Brown 1992; Schelhas 1994). In the context of an analysis of a proposed prospecting program, decision makers may need to identify a preferred alternative based on estimates of all other direct and indirect benefits and then qualitatively consider whether the existence value associated with preserving biodiversity is cause for some modification of this decision.

Quasi-Option Value

Another important consideration involved in conservation planning is the value of maintaining the opportunity to benefit from a protected site if biochemical prospecting opportunities or other services provided by the natural ecosystem become more valuable in the future. This type of contingent benefit of ecosystem preservation is referred to by some authors as quasi-option value and by others simply as option value (Weisbrod 1964; Arrow and Fisher 1974; Henry 1974; Fisher and Haneman 1986). To differentiate it from the related but distinct valuation concepts developed in the literature on financial options, I will refer to the benefit of delaying irreversible habitat conversion as quasi-option value. The relationship between the quasi-option value of habitat preservation and the value of an option to perform biochemical prospecting is discussed in more detail in the last section of this chapter.

Arrow and Fisher (1974) and Fisher and Hanneman (1986) have shown that if new information is expected to become available, there is a positive value associated with making current choices that preserve the option to utilize that information. With continued improvements in technologies for screening biological extracts, as well as advances in ecological and biochemical knowledge, even an ecosystem that has already been the focus of biochemical prospecting efforts could be the source of valuable biochemical discoveries in the future. It is quite possible that, in addition to changes in the value of biochemical resources, changing conditions could increase the value of ecotourism or environmental services provided by the preserved ecosystem. Changing moral perspectives on environmental protection could also lead to increases in existence value over time. Ideally, judgments regarding the probability of future values of all of these variables should be incorporated into the evaluation of quasi-option value. By deciding to postpone ecologically destructive development, the host government leaves open the option of obtaining the benefits of biochemical prospecting, ecotourism, and environmental services from that area in the future.

A common approach used in project analysis is to translate uncertain benefits and costs into expected values and then to choose the alternative with the maximum expected net benefits. However, a decision to convert a biologically rich ecosystem to some other land-use could lead to the extinction of many locally endemic species. As a result, the option of screening biochemical samples of these species for their potential commercial value would be permanently eliminated. If the decision to develop or preserve a natural area can be postponed until new information (e.g., new screening technologies, additional ecological knowledge, changes in market prices) is received, then a correctly specified decision analysis would include a calculation of the expected maximum benefits of the economic opportunities that will be available in the future, given current land-use choices.

With respect to the quasi-option value associated with biochemical prospecting, the host government should be most concerned with how new information might affect the value and number of species that are not adequately protected at other sites within the country. The number of species known to be in this category might increase over time due to new ecological research at the prospecting location or extinction of local populations at other sites. New medical research, as well as the continued evolution of drug-resistant diseases, might increase the value of screening extracts from these species. In addition, the host country's technological development may eventually enable it to capture a larger share of the benefits of biochemical prospecting projects. Incorporating these considerations into a simple numerical example may provide an improved understanding of quasi-option value.

Consider a relatively pristine natural area that could be the site of a biochemical prospecting effort or could be converted to some incompatible agricultural or industrial use. Conversion of the site would cause an estimated 100 species endemic to the area to become extinct. The expected net present value of benefits from conversion are $1.0 million in Period 1 and $1.0 million in Period 2. Total net benefits of preservation in Period 1 are $0.8 million. However, second-period benefits of preservation depend on the results of ongoing ecological and biomedical research. Assume there is a 50 percent chance of depreciation in the present value of preservation to $0.4 million in Period 2 and a 50 percent chance that new information will cause the present value of preserving the site's biodiversity during the second period to appreciate to $1.6 million. For simplicity, also assume that in Period 1 the site must be either completely developed or completely preserved. If the site is preserved in Period 1 but the second-period value of preservation has declined, conversion to the alternative use can still occur in Period 2.

In this problem, the expected present value of conversion is $2.0 million, while the expected present value of preservation over both periods is $1.8 million.[3] If the decision maker were to select a single land-use for both periods by comparing the expected net present value of benefits of each land-use, this would lead to conversion of the site and extinction of an estimated 100 species in Period 1. However, since new information about the benefits of preservation will be available at the start of Period 2, the correct decision rule would be to maximize the total of first-period benefits plus the expected best choice available in Period 2 after the new information becomes available. If the site is preserved in Period 1, then the host country retains the option of continuing to preserve the site in Period 2 or proceeding with conversion to an alternative land-use. Given the assumptions that were made about how new information could affect second-period benefits, the correct calculation of the expected value of preservation is therefore:

$0.8 million + (.5 x $1.6 million) + (.5 x $1.0 million) = $2.1 million

By incorporating the expected value of new information into the decision, preservation in Period 1 becomes the appropriate choice. This decision problem is represented graphically in Figure 3.3.

$$Q = BP_t|\Theta_{t-1} + \xi_t - \sum_{t=1}^{T} \sum_{\Theta t} \{[p(\Theta_t)|\Theta_{t-1}]BP_t|\Theta_{t-1}\} \qquad (3.3)$$

For a multiperiod, binary choice between complete preservation or complete conversion, quasi-option value can be defined more rigorously as follows.[4] Let Θ_t be a random variable that represents the possible combinations of new information that could be received during time t (e.g., in terms of the estimated number of species endemic to the prospecting site and the value of each sample obtained from these endemic species), let $p(\Theta_t)|\Theta_{t-1}$ indicate the probability of information state Θ_t, given the occurrence of information state Θ_{t-1}, let $BP_t|\Theta_{t-1}$ be the present value of the benefits of preservation in period t given Θ_{t-1}, let BC_t be the present value of the benefits of conversion in period t, and let T be the terminal period of the analysis. Then quasi-option value can be computed using the recursive equation shown below:[5]

where

$$\xi_t = \sum_{\Theta t} p(\Theta_t)|\Theta_{t-1} \max[BP_{t+1}| \Theta_t + \xi_{t+1}, \sum_{i=t+1}^{T} BC_i] \qquad (3.3a)$$

and

$$\text{and } \xi_T = 0 \qquad\qquad (3.3b)$$

Quasi-option value as defined in Equation 3.3 can be summarized as the difference between the expected value of preservation when the potential for future changes in land-use are included in the analysis and the expected value of preservation when these future economic options are not taken into account.

Fisher and Hanemann (1986) provide a simple proof indicating that in a binary choice where one alternative involves irreversible consequences, quasi-option value must be nonnegative. This does not mean that preservation is always the correct choice. In the simple example presented above, if the maximum second-period value of preservation were only $13 million instead of $16 million, then conversion would be the appropriate decision in Period 1 even when the potential effects of new information are taken into account. What the positive sign of quasi-option value does indicate is that, since species extinction is irreversible and new technologies and scientific discoveries may increase the value of biodiversity, greater efforts should be made to preserve biodiversity than might be justified by its current or expected value.

Despite Fisher and Hanemann's proof, there has been some confusion in the economic literature over both the sign and the importance of quasi-option value. Some commentators have mistakenly assumed that since new information can increase or decrease the value of preservation, quasi-option value can be both positive and negative and is therefore not a critical factor in conservation decisions (Freeman 1984; Aylward 1992, p. 425). One point about which there is general agreement in the literature is that quasi-option value does not represent a distinct category of benefits (Fisher and Hanemann 1987; Freeman 1984). Net benefits computed as part of a properly specified decision analysis will necessarily include quasi-option value. In terms of the analysis of a proposed prospecting contract, the effects of current choices on future economic opportunities given probable future states of the world should be explicitly considered, as described in the numerical example on page 76 and depicted graphically in Figure 3.3.

FIGURE 3.3. Two-Period, Binary Land-Use Decision with Irreversible Conversion Alternative

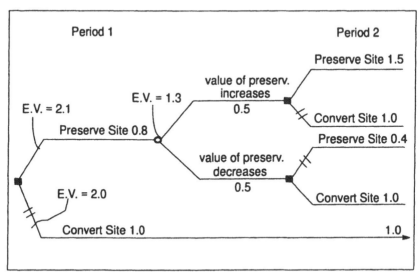

In theory, the decision analysis of whether to preserve or convert a natural ecosystem should include the interaction among land-use choices, new information, and changes in economic factors over an infinite time horizon. In most cases, however, this kind of infinite horizon analysis would be not only impractical but also unnecessary. If the host country's discount rate is relatively high, then the value of preserving future options would decline rapidly as those options become more distant in time. In addition, benefits from biochemical prospecting and alternate land-uses may not be expected to shift significantly and durably over very short periods of time. In this case, a simplified multiperiod analysis, with each time period consisting of five or ten years, might be sufficient to reflect the essential factors of the land-use decision confronting the host country.

In addition to conversion of the prospecting location(s) to other land-uses, the host country also has the option of refusing the prospecting opportunity but leaving the prospecting locations undisturbed. One scenario where the host country might preserve the sight but refuse the prospecting offer is if the proposed contract granted some degree of exclusive prospecting rights for a significant period of time at an unreasonably low price. Alternatively, the proposed contract might limit the host country's options to utilize the prospecting locations for other economic activities in the future. These considerations again highlight the importance of a multiperiod decision analysis that includes the economic opportunities available both during and after the proposed contract.

A final consideration regarding the interaction between biochemical prospecting and quasi-option value involves the potential benefits of information generated by the prospecting effort. To the degree that the prospecting contract yields new biogeographical, ecological, or biochemical information; new species collection techniques; or more highly trained scientists and technicians, the host country may be better equipped to negotiate, conduct, and benefit from future prospecting efforts. It may also have obtained important information with which to identify and avoid unprofitable prospecting opportunities in the future. In general, a biochemical prospecting contract that involves significant participation on the part of the host country is likely to result in valuable information and skills that will alter the expected benefits of future prospecting opportunities relative to a decision path that declined the prospecting opportunity.

Summarizing the Analysis and Incorporating Risk Aversion

The preceding discussion indicates that an analytical framework for evaluating proposed biochemical prospecting contracts must be able to incorporate both site-specific prospecting efforts as well as prospecting contracts that require collection of extracts from numerous locations within the country. In addition, the analysis must be flexible enough to evaluate a variety of other potential uses for the prospecting location(s) that may result in various degrees of alteration of the natural ecosystem. It is also important to incorporate estimates of amenity and existence values into the analysis if the prospecting contract is being compared with land-use options that require conversion of the natural ecosystem. Finally, the potential effect of new information and changes in economic variables should be taken into account through a multiperiod decision model that considers the effect of current decisions on the options available to the host country in the future. The essential elements of the analysis are summarized in Figure 3.4.

If the biochemical prospecting project involves only a small fraction of the host country's economic assets, the decision analysis can be conducted primarily in terms of expected monetary benefits using a risk-free discount rate (Arrow 1963). Yet even without adding any additional risk premium, a developing country's discount rate may be quite high given the current need to satisfy basic needs of its population.

If the biochemical prospecting project requires a sizable commitment of the host country's land, capital, or technical talent, then potential monetary costs and benefits cannot simply be translated into expected values. One common response to this problem is to use a discount rate for the evaluation of each alternative that reflects the expected returns on other, similarly risky investments. For example, if the returns from agriculture are less variable than those from pharmaceutical R&D, the host country might use a lower, risk-adjusted discount rate for evaluation of the alternative of agricultural conversion than for the alternative of proceeding with the biochemical prospecting effort. The problem with this approach is that it does not separate the effects of time preference from those of risk aversion, potentially leading to inappropriate decisions.

A more theoretically appropriate method for treating risk-averse preferences is to derive a utility function for the decision maker that relates any given amount of monetary gain or loss with a unique level of utility (Luce and Raiffa 1957). As shown in Figure 3.5, a utility function for a risk-averse decision maker would be concave, indicating that the value of each unit increase in monetary gain declines as the level of monetary returns increases.

Given an appropriate utility function for the host country, it would be possible to evaluate each alternative in the decision analysis in terms of its expected utility as opposed to its expected monetary value. The necessary steps in the analysis would be to apply a risk-neutral discount rate to calculate the net present monetary value of each potential outcome, use the host country's utility function to compute the utility of each monetary outcome, and then conduct the decision analysis using these utility values. Methods for estimating the potential

FIGURE 3.4. Summary of Host Country Decision Analysis

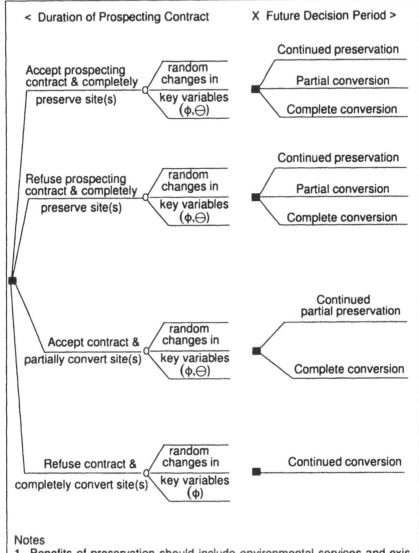

Notes
1. Benefits of preservation should include environmental services and existence value when compared with conversion of natural ecosystem(s).
2. Current land-use choices affect future options.
3. Information gained from prospecting contract or partial conversion of site(s) may increase expected benefits of future land-use/economic options.

FIGURE 3.5. Sample Utility Function

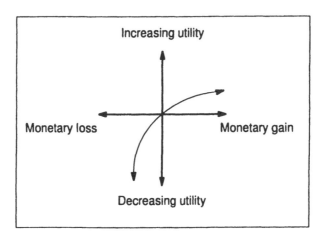

variability in returns from a biochemical prospecting program and techniques for comparing the utility of various contractual alternatives are discussed in more detail in the next chapter.

In practice, a small group of government officials, academic researchers, and business leaders are likely to be responsible for evaluating proposed prospecting contracts and conducting contract negotiations. Ideally, their choices should reflect the risk preferences of the people whose interests they are purporting to represent. However, there is likely to be a divergence between the risks and rewards of a biochemical prospecting endeavor for these decision makers and for the general populace of the host country.

Integrating Biochemical Prospecting Opportunities into Land-Use Planning

Due to population growth and continued conversion of natural habitats, conservation strategies must increasingly focus on preserving biodiversity as part of a complex mosaic of modified and natural ecosystems. As a result, guidelines for nature reserve planning and management have begun to incorporate insights gained from landscape ecology and studies of habitat fragmentation (Margules, Nicoll, and Pressey 1988; Saunder, Hobbs, and Margules 1991; Hunter 1991; Scott et al. 1991). However, except for an occasional acknowledgment of the constraints posed by political and economic realities, these guidelines generally have not explicitly included economic criteria.

The bioeconomic approach to land-use planning presented below is an extension of the decision theoretic framework presented earlier in this chapter. However, in this extended model, there is no presumption that a specific prospecting proposal is under consideration. Rather, it is assumed that there is an existing market for biological samples or extracts. Expected net revenues from collection and sale of biological material are evaluated as one of the benefits of preservation. Depending on the limits of the computational resources available, the model can include any number of potential prospecting locations, varying degrees of preservation at each site, and multiple time periods.

In its broadest application, the expanded analytical approach presented in this section can be used to consider the issue of how much of a country's representative ecosystems should be preserved. A smaller-scale application might be to determine which of the remnants of one or more ecosystem types should be designated as nature reserves. The model is not intended to provide definitive answers regarding the optimum level of conservation. Given the rudimentary state of knowledge in conservation biology and landscape ecology and the difficulty of estimating the economic value of environmental resources, such a goal would be unrealistic and misleading. Nevertheless, countries must continually make decisions, whether explicit or implicit, regarding the preservation of natural ecosystems relative to competing land-uses. The analytical framework presented below has been designed to utilize available information, to permit easy incorporation of new data as it is generated, and to provide a means to evaluate the benefits of obtaining new information prior to making irreversible decisions.

The analysis of land-use decisions at many sites or ecosystems over time can be depicted graphically as a decision tree or can be represented mathematically in the form of a dynamic programming problem. If the analysis involves more than a very few sites, time periods, land-use choices, and stochastic events, the graphical presentation can quickly become unwieldy. However, as the number of possible combinations of locations, land-use choices, time periods, and states of the world is increased, the "curse of dimensionality" begins to impair

even a computer-aided dynamic programming analysis. With this caution in mind, I will present the planning problem first in a generalized
form and then illustrate it by way of a simple example.

Let A_0 be a vector indicating the preserved area in each of L locations at time $t = 0$. Let P_t and C_t be vectors indicating the proportion of
each location preserved in its natural state at the start of period t and
the proportion of each location irreversibly converted to other land-
uses during period t. Let $f(A_0, P_t, C_t, \Phi_t)$ indicate the benefits derived
in period t from converted land as a (decreasing) function of the degree
of preservation in each ecosystem at the start of period t, the degree of
conversion during period t, and the random variable Φ_t. Let $g(A_0, P_t,
C_t, \Theta_t)$ indicate the benefits of preservation in period t as a function of
the degree of preservation in each ecosystem at the start of period t, the
degree of conversion during period t, and a random variable Θ_t. Let
$P_{i,t}$ and $C_{i,t}$ indicate the degree of preservation at the start of period t
and the degree of conversion during period t at location i. Finally, let δ
be the effective discount rate for each period. If the host country's
objective is to maximize the present value of benefits derived from
converted and preserved land over the time period $t = 0$ to T, the
objective function can be defined as follows:

$$\underset{C_t}{\text{Max}}\ TB = \sum_{t=0}^{T} (1+\delta)^{-t}[f(A_0, P_t, C_t, \Phi_t) + g(A_0, P_t, C_t, \Theta_t)] \quad (3.4)$$

$$\text{s.t. } P_{i,t+1} = P_{i,t} - C_{i,t}\ \forall i \quad (3.4a)$$

$$0 \le C_{i,t} \le P_{i,t} \le 1\ \forall i \quad (3.4b)$$

The recursive equation for this stochastic dynamic programming
problem is shown below:

$$TB_t^*(A_0, P_t, \Phi_t, \Theta_t) = \underset{C_t}{\text{Max}}\,[f(A_0, P_t, C_t, \Phi_{t-1}) + g(A_0, P_t, C_t, \Theta_{t-1})]+$$

$$\underset{\Phi_t \Theta_t}{\sum\sum} p(\Phi_t | \Phi_{t-1})\ p(\Theta_t | \Theta_{t-1}) TB_{t+1}^*(A_0, P_{t+1}, C_{t+1}, \Phi_t, \Theta_t)(1+\delta)^{-1}$$

$$(3.5)$$

subject to the same constraints as in Equation 3.4 and where $p(\Phi_t|\Phi_{t-1})$ and $p(\Theta_t|\Theta_{t-1})$ represent the probability that a particular value of Φ_t or Θ_t will occur given the occurrence of particular values of Φ_{t-1} and Θ_{t-1}, respectively.[6]

To develop a more intuitive understanding of the problem summarized by Equations 3.4 and 3.5, it may be useful to present a simple application. Suppose the host country is developing land-use plans for two ecosystems or locations ($L = 2$), and the possible land-use choices for each ecosystem are limited to total preservation, preservation of two-thirds of the ecosystem, preservation of one-third, and total conversion. At the start of Period 1, there are 16 possible combinations of land-use choices, each of which can be represented by the state vector P_t. For example (0,0) indicates complete conversion of both ecosystems; (0,.33) indicates complete conversion of Ecosystem 1 and preservation of one-third of Ecosystem 2; (.33,.67) indicates preservation of one-third of Ecosystem 1 and two-thirds of Ecosystem 2; etc. To permit a relatively simple graphical representation of the problem, I shall assume that the host country is developing land-use plans for a two-period time horizon and that the values of Φ_1 and Φ_2 are known with certainty at the start of Period 1. The value of Θ_1 is also known at the start of Period 1, but the value of Θ_2 will not be known until the start of Period 2. I have also assumed that relative to Θ_1, the value of Θ_2 could increase by 100 percent or decrease by 50 percent with equal probability. This decision problem is depicted graphically in Figure 3.6.

By completely converting both sites in Period 1, the host country eliminates any preservation options in Period 2, regardless of the value of preservation. At the other extreme, choosing to completely preserve both ecosystems in Period 1 preserves the option of selecting the most beneficial of the 16 possible land-use combinations in Period 2, given the revealed value of Θ_2. Complete preservation in Period 1 allows the host country to obtain the full benefit of the information conveyed by changes in Θ_t. First-period land-use choices that lie between the extremes of complete conversion and complete preservation permit the host country to obtain some of the value of new information, since these partial preservation alternatives maintain some—but not all—second-period land-use options, as illustrated by the decision tree in Figure 3.6.[7]

FIGURE 3.6. Partial Decision Tree for Two-Period, Two-Location Land-Use Planning Problem

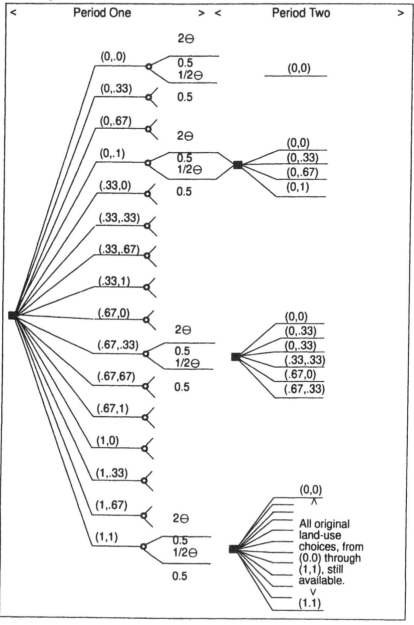

Additional insights can be gained by adding some numerical detail to this hypothetical land-use planning problem. Assume that the benefits of conversion, denominated in thousands of dollars, can be represented by the following function:

$$BC_t = \varkappa 1[A_{1,0}(1-P_{1,t}+C_{1,t})]^{\alpha 1} + \varkappa 2[A_{2,0}(1-P_{2,t} + C_{2,t})]^{\alpha 2} \quad (3.6)$$

$$0 \le C_{1,t} \le P_{1,t} \le 1 \quad\quad (3.6a)$$

$$0 \le C_{2,t} \le P_{2,t} \le 1 \quad\quad (3.6b)$$

$$P_{1,t+1} = P_{1,t} - C_{1,t} \quad\quad (3.6c)$$

$$P_{2,t+1} = P_{2,t} - C_{2,t} \quad\quad (3.6d)$$

where $A_{1,0}$ and $A_{2,0}$ are the original areas of Ecosystems 1 and 2 in square kilometers, $P_{1,t}$ and $P_{2,t}$ are the proportions of the original area of each ecosystem that are still preserved at the start of period t, $C_{1,t}$ and $C_{2,t}$ are the proportions of each ecosystem converted to other uses during period t, and $\varkappa 1$, $\varkappa 2$, $\alpha 1$ and $\alpha 2$ are constants that reflect the initial and marginal productivity of conversion.[8]

The benefits of preservation, excluding those derived from biochemical prospecting, are summarized by the following equation:

$$BE_t = \lambda 1[A_{1,0}(P_{1,t}-C_{1,t})]^{\beta 1} + \lambda 2[A_{2,0}(P_{2,t}-C_{2,t})]^{\beta 2} \quad (3.7)$$

which is subject to the same constraints as Equation 3.6, and where $\lambda 1$, $\lambda 2$, $\beta 1$, and $\beta 2$ are constants reflecting the initial and marginal productivity of preservation.

The net benefit received by the host country from biochemical prospecting is the difference between the total compensation received for biological extracts or samples and the cost of collecting and preparing them.[9] The first difficulty in estimating this net benefit function is determining the value of each biological sample. Differences in the demand for samples of microorganisms, plants, insects, and other animals may justify analyzing each of these markets separately. Using the analytical framework described in the following chapter, the host country could determine the guaranteed payments that are equivalent to the expected utility of the total compensation package likely to be offered in exchange for samples from each of these categories.[10] It is these utility equivalent guaranteed payments, or certainty equivalents, that should be used as the market values (v) of samples from each category.

Given a market value for samples or extracts from each category, the host country must still estimate the marginal cost of producing them. With this information it can then determine the optimal level of production and the expected net benefit from biochemical prospecting. Although an informal market for biological extracts has operated for some time, I am not aware of any country, prospecting organization, or scientific organization that has developed empirical data on the costs of systematically collecting samples from a substantial portion of the species in a particular ecosystem.[11] In the absence of such data, I will rely on a few simple observations to develop a cost function. First, it would be expected that the marginal cost of collecting each sample would increase as the number of unsampled species decreases. In addition, after samples have been collected from virtually all of the species of interest in the ecosystem or prospecting location, the marginal cost of obtaining samples from the last one or two species could be nearly infinite. Something quite similar to finding a needle in a haystack. A marginal collection cost function of the following form displays these two characteristics:

$$MC(N) = k\frac{S}{S-N} \tag{3.8}$$

where S is the total number of species of interest, N is the number of species from which samples have been collected, and k is a constant equivalent to the cost of collecting and preparing the first sample. The total cost of collecting N samples is therefore the integral of $MC(N)$, over the range 0 to N.

$$TC(N) = \int_{n=0}^{N} k\frac{S}{S-n} \, dn = [-\ln(S-n)kS] \, \Big|_0^N \tag{3.9}$$

Since the cost of collecting and preparing samples is also likely to differ across taxonomic groups, a more detailed analysis might utilize different market values and collection cost functions for plants, insects, microorganisms, and larger animals. Collection costs and market values also might differ for previously identified species relative to undiscovered ones. However, for purposes of this example, I shall continue with the analysis in the context of a single market price and collection cost function.

Given a market value for each extract and a collection cost function, the host country's problem is to determine the number of samples to collect and sell to maximize its net benefits.[12] This maximization problem is defined below:

$$\underset{N}{Max}\ BP = vN + \int_{n=0}^{N} k\frac{S}{S-n}\,dn \tag{3.10}$$

$$0 \leq N \leq S \tag{3.10a}$$

Assuming that the cost of obtaining the first sample is less than its market value, the host country can maximize the net benefit from prospecting by continuing to collect samples until the marginal benefit, v, equals the marginal cost, $MC(N)$. Setting marginal cost equal to marginal benefit and solving for N yields the optimal number of extracts or samples to collect:

$$v = k\frac{S}{S-N_{opt}} \Rightarrow N_{opt} = S\left(1-\frac{k}{v}\right) \tag{3.11}$$

Substituting N_{opt} into Equation 2.10 yields the potential net benefits of prospecting as a function of the number of species in the ecosystem and the market value of each biological sample:

$$BP_{opt} = vS\left(1-\frac{k}{v}\right) - \int_{n=0}^{S\left(1-\frac{k}{v}\right)} k\left(\frac{S}{S-n}\right)\,dn \tag{3.12}$$

which can be simplified to

$$BP_{opt} = S\left[v-k-k\ln\left(\frac{v}{k}\right)\right] \tag{3.13}$$

Equation 3.13 provides an estimate of the maximum expected benefits that can be obtained by selling biological samples obtained from an ecosystem with S marketable species, given a particular form for the collection cost function. But the choice variables in the land-use planning example that I have been developing are the amounts of land to preserve at each location. Therefore, Equation 3.13 must be restated as a function of the land area in a given

ecosystem or potential prospecting location. The species-area relationship derived from the theory of island biogeography provides
one basis for this restatement.

Island biogeography theory predicts that the number of species in
an ecosystem is an increasing function of the size of the ecosystem.
The mathematical relationship between number of species and ecosystem size is referred to as a species-area curve. Although there is
significant controversy over the biological basis and potential
implications of this relationship, species-area curves are often used
to predict the number of species that will be lost in a given ecosystem due to land conversion (Myers 1988; Wilson 1988; Lovejoy
1980; Simberloff 1986; Raven 1988; Reid 1992). There is no single
functional form of the species-area curve that provides the best fit
of the data from a wide range of ecosystems. The most commonly
used form is the power curve shown below (Simberloff 1992):

$$S = \gamma A^z \qquad\qquad (3.14)$$

where A is the area of the ecosystem and γ and z are fitted constants.
Empirical studies have found that for most ecosystems the value of
z lies between 0.15 and 0.4 (Connor and McCoy 1979). The higher
the value of z, the steeper the species-area curve.

Substituting Equation 3.14 into Equation 3.13 provides an estimate
of the benefits of biochemical prospecting as a function of the land
area of the ecosystem and the market value of biological samples.

$$BP_{opt} = \gamma A^z \left[v - k - k \ln\left(\frac{v}{k}\right) \right] \qquad\qquad (3.15)$$

In the context of decisions about whether to extend some form of
protected status to currently unprotected natural areas, the estimate
of the biochemical prospecting value of an ecosystem, summarized
in Equation 2.15, must be revised to account for the existence of
some species at more than one location. Once a species has been
protected in one ecosystem, the marginal benefit of preserving its
habitat at another location will be reduced. It would therefore be
appropriate to focus primarily on those species that are not adequately protected at other sites within the country (Scott et al.
1991). In addition, if the host country is attempting to determine

what degree or extent of protection to provide to several currently unprotected sites, then the overlap between species found at these sites must also be considered. Unfortunately, even if good data exist on the distribution of species between sites in the analysis, it is difficult to predict how these relationships will be affected by land conversion at one or more sites.

If it is assumed that partial site conversion will have proportionately the same effect on locally unique species and on species found at more than one site, some general adjustment for species overlap becomes possible.[13] But even with this simplifying assumption, the analysis can quickly become unwieldy or require data that are unlikely to be available. The following is an attempt to account for species overlap between sites in a manner that seeks to balance accuracy and computational simplicity, while keeping in mind the meager information normally available on species distribution in many ecosystems.

I shall define overlapping species to be those species which are not abundant or adequately protected at other sites within the country but which can be found at one or more locations included in the land-use planning analysis. Let L be the number of locations in the analysis, let $S_{i,t}$ be the number of species at location i at time t, let ϵ_i be the proportion of all species at location i that are overlapping species, let r_{ij} be the proportion of overlapping species at location i that can also be found at location j at time $t = 0$, and let r_{iL} be the proportion of overlapping species at location I that can also be found at time $t = 0$ at one or more other locations included in the analysis.[14] Finally, let the dynamic additive correlation between sites be defined as follows:

$$R_{i,t} = \left(\sum_{j=1}^{L} \frac{r_{ij} S_{j,t}}{S_{j,0}} \right) - \frac{S_{i,t}}{S_{i,0}} \qquad (3.16)$$

and substituting the species area curve for S yields

$$R_{i,t} = \left[\sum_{j=1}^{L} \frac{r_{ij} \epsilon_j \gamma_j [A_{j,0}(P_{j,t} - C_{j,t})]^{z_j}}{\epsilon_j \gamma_j A_{j,0}^{z_j}} \right] - \frac{\epsilon_i \gamma_i [A_{i,0}(P_{i,t} - C_{i,t})]^{z_i}}{\epsilon_i \gamma_i A_{i,0}^{z_i}} \qquad (3.17)$$

Given these definitions, the benefits of biochemical prospecting in L ecosystems can be approximated as follows to take account of the presence of species at multiple locations:

$$\underset{N_i^*}{Max\ BP_t} = \sum_{i=1}^{L} \left[v_t N_i - \int_{n=0}^{N_i^*} k_j \frac{\left(1 - \frac{r_{i_L} R_{i,t}}{R_{i,t}+r_{i_L}}\right) \varepsilon_i \gamma_i A_{i,0}^{z_i}}{\left(1 - \frac{r_{i_L} R_{i,t}}{R_{i,t}+r_{i_L}}\right) \varepsilon_i \gamma_i A_{i,0}^{z_i} - n} dn \right] \tag{3.18}$$

$$s.t.\ 0 \le N_i < \left(1 - \frac{r_{iL} R_{i,t}}{R_{i,t}+r_{i_L}}\right) \varepsilon_i \gamma_i A_{i,0}^{z_i}$$

Assuming the cost of collecting the first sample is less than its market value and the cost of collecting a sample from every species would exceed the market value, the solution to this maximization problem can again be found by selecting each N_i such that the marginal cost of collecting biological samples in each of the locations is equivalent to the marginal benefit. These conditions are defined below:

$$v_t = k_j \frac{\left(1 - \frac{r_{i_L} R_{i,t}}{R_{i,t}+r_{i_L}}\right) \varepsilon_i \gamma_i A_{i,0}^{z_i}}{\left(1 - \frac{r_{i_L} R_{i,t}}{R_{i,t}+r_{i_L}}\right) \varepsilon_i \gamma_i A_{i,0}^{z_i} - N_i}\ \forall i \tag{3.19}$$

Solving for N_i yields the optimal number of samples to collect from each ecosystem, as shown below:

$$N_i^* = \varepsilon_i \gamma_i A_{i,0}^{z_i} \left(1 - \frac{r_{iL} R_{i,t}}{R_{i,t}+r_{i_L}}\right)\left(1 - \frac{k_j}{v_t}\right) \tag{3.20}$$

Substituting N_i^* into Equation 3.18 and simplifying yields the following equation for the biochemical prospecting value of several ecosystems with overlapping species.

$$BP_t^* = \sum_{i=1}^{L} \varepsilon_i \gamma_i A_{i,0}^{z_i} \left(1 - \frac{r_{iL} R_{i,t}}{R_{i,t}+r_{i_L}}\right)\left[v_t - k_j - k_j \ln\left(\frac{v_t}{k_j}\right)\right] \tag{3.21}$$

The foregoing adjustment for species overlap is far from ideal. For example, if more than two ecosystems are included in the analysis, the algorithm presented above tends to underestimate species overlap for land-use configurations that involve disproportionate habitat conversion for a subset of the ecosystems in the analysis. Still, the adjusted equations provide more accurate results than a system of equations, which does not account for species overlap at all.[15] In addition, the above procedure for incorporating species overlap has the considerable advantage of requiring relatively simple data that are likely to be available for many ecosystems.

Determining the present value of biochemical prospecting benefits is further complicated by the potential for changes in market prices. An increase in the market value of biological samples would increase the optimal number of samples to collect and presumably increase the collection rate. In addition, after a sample has tested negatively for one or more potential uses, its market value should be lower than a sample from an untested species. As the period of time since a species was screened for potential chemical value increases, the price differential relative to samples from previously unscreened species is likely to diminish.

For purposes of the two-period, two-location land-use planning example, I have assumed that the value of each sample (v_t), is fixed during each time period, and collection of the optimal number of samples, given v_t, occurs evenly throughout each time period. At the start of Period 1, v_1 is known, and no samples have been collected or tested from either ecosystem. It is also assumed that samples from a species are tested for biochemical value only once during each time period.[16] The uncertain effect of changes in technology and other factors is incorporated into the analysis through random changes in the market value of samples (both tested and untested) at the start of the second period. More specifically, the second period market value of a sample, v_2, is the product of v_1 and the random variable $\ominus_2$, which is assumed to take on values of 2.0 and 0.5 with equal probability. Since development of new technologies for biological screening and manipulation, the evolution of drug-resistant strains of existing diseases, and the emergence of new diseases would all tend to create renewed demand for samples from species that have already been tested, no differential is assumed to exist between the market value of a sample from a previously uncollected species and a sample from a species that was tested during the previous period.

Combining the benefit functions for biochemical prospecting, ecosystem preservation and conversion with the relevant constraints, and random variables yields the following two-period maximization problem:

$$\underset{c1,c2_1}{Max}\ TB_1 = BC_1 + BE_1 + BP^*_1 + .5[TB_2|(\ominus_2 = 2)] + .5[TB_2|(\ominus_2 = .5)]$$

$$s.t.\ 0 \le C1_t, C2_t, P1_t, P2_t \le 1\ and\ C1_t \le P1_t\ and\ C2_t \le P2_t$$

$$(3.22)$$

Summary results for this two-period, two-location dynamic programming example are depicted in Figure 3.7, with the full computational detail presented in Appendix B. Location 1 could be thought of as a large, relatively undisturbed ecosystem, and Location 2 as the much smaller remnant of what was once a similarly expansive natural ecosystem. In Ecosystem 2, the more fertile and profitable land has already been converted to other uses. Therefore, the marginal return to land conversion is lower, and the marginal benefits of preservation (e.g., watershed protection, ecotourism) are higher in Location 2 than in the larger and relatively unconverted Location 1. In addition, the proportion of species endemic to Location 2 is greater than in Location 1.

Given the specific numerical assumptions summarized in Figure 3.7, the optimal land-use decision in Period 1 is to preserve one-third of Ecosystem 1 and all of Ecosystem 2. In Period 2, the optimal land-use decision will depend on the revealed value of biological samples in Period 2. If the value of biological samples doubles, optimal land-use in Period 2 would be to continue to preserve all previously unconverted land (i.e., $P_2 = .33,1$). If the value of biological samples declines by 50 percent, optimal land-use in Period 2 would be to preserve the remainder of Ecosystem 1 and convert one-third of Ecosystem 2 ($P_2 = .33,.67$).

Obviously, the model outlined above does not incorporate many of the social and political complexities of conservation and land-use planning in developing countries. The strengths of the model are its ability to incorporate a range of economic values and numerous sites while simplifying the policy choice variables to the amount of preserved area. The analysis can be performed for more than two time periods and a range of possible values for the future market

FIGURE 3.7. Summary of Results for Sample Land-Use Planning Problem

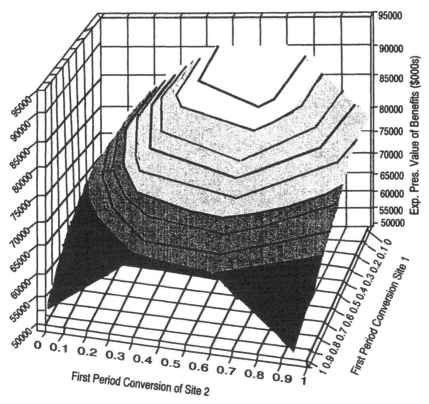

Max PVB = for t = 1 to 2Σ [$BC_t + BE_t + BP_t / (1+\delta)^{t-1}$] s.t. $0 \leq P_{1,t}, P_{2,t}, C_{1,t}, C_{2,t} \leq 1$

$BC = \varkappa_1 [A_1 (P_{1,t} - C_{1,t})]^{\alpha 1} + \varkappa_2 [A_2 (P_{2,t} - C_{2,t})]^{\alpha 2}$ $BE = \lambda_1[A_1 (P_{1,t} - C_{1,t})] \beta^1 + \lambda_2 [A_2(P_{2,t} - C_{2,t})] \beta^2$

BP = for 1 = 1 to 2 $\Sigma \{\varepsilon_1\gamma_1 (A_1)^{Z_i}[1-r_{iL}R_{i,t} /(R_{i,t}+r_{iL})] \} [v_t - k_i - k_i\ln (v_t / k_i)]\}$

where $R_{i,t}$ = for j = 1 to 2 $\Sigma \{r_{ij}\varepsilon_j\gamma_j[A_j(P_{j,t} - C_{j,t}Z_j] / \varepsilon_j\gamma_j(A_j)^{Z_j}\} - \varepsilon_i\gamma_i[A_i(P_{i,t} - C_{i,t})^{Z_i}] /\varepsilon_i\gamma_i(A_i)^{Z_i}$

A_1 = 10,000	$\varkappa_1$ = 100	$\alpha 1$ = 0.4	λ_1 = 20	r_{12} = 0.20	e_1 = 0.5
A_2 = 1,000	$\varkappa_2$ = 75	α_2 = 0.3	λ_2 = 30	r_{21} = 0.45	e_2 = 0.7
γ_1 = 5,000	Z_1 = 0.35	β_1 = 0.5	k_1 = 100	r_{1L} = 0.20	δ = 0.05
γ_2 = 5,000	Z_2 = 0.35	β_2 = 0.6	k_2 = 75	r_{2L} = 0.45	v_1 = \$300
v_2 = \$150 or \$600 with equal probability				Years per period = 10	

price of biological resources. In fact, any of the parameters in the analysis that affect the benefits of conversion, preservation, or prospecting can be treated as uncertain variables with a probability distribution over a range of values. This enables the decision maker to estimate the benefits of obtaining additional information on the true value of these parameters prior to making any long-term or irreversible land-use decisions. Several methods for generating additional information on the benefits of biochemical prospecting are discussed in following sections of this chapter.

Further refinements of the model might involve developing a benefit function for biochemical prospecting that involves not only the amount but also the pattern of preserved land within each ecosystem. It is generally acknowledged that the degree of fragmentation within an ecosystem and the types of land-uses surrounding a natural area will significantly affect the number and types of species that will survive within it (Janzen 1986; Lovejoy et al. 1986). In addition, extinction of endemic animal and plant populations due to partial conversion of a natural ecosystem usually occurs gradually over time, and in some cases, population declines can be arrested or reversed through ecological restoration efforts (Simberloff 1992; Heywood and Stuart 1992). Incorporating this temporal aspect of the species-area affect would tend to minimize the quasi-option value of ecosystem preservation.

STRATEGIES FOR SUSTAINABLE DEVELOPMENT OF BIOLOGICAL RESOURCES

National Policies and Legal Systems

A favorable national policy environment is a key ingredient for the development of any new industry. With regard to biochemical prospecting and related biochemical research and processing activities, the minimal elements of a supportive national policy environment include effective programs for biodiversity conservation, legislation defining access and real property rights, and effective protection of intellectual property rights.

It is difficult to envision sustainable development of biological resources if the resource itself is in rapid decline. Without effective protection of biodiversity, long-term investments to extract economic profits from these resources will not be forthcoming. Some ex-situ collection and screening activity may be pursued, but the risks of natural product research are much greater if the species from which samples have been obtained cannot be studied and recollected in situ. The existence of a system of public and privately owned areas that are in fact truly protected is a prerequisite for creation of a significant biochemical prospecting program.

Protection of biodiversity must be accompanied by clear guidelines that define how to legally obtain access to it for purposes of commercial research and development. This requires the definition of national, communal, and individual property rights over biochemical extracts and genetic material derived from plant and animal species and creation of a permit system for biochemical prospecting activities. At one extreme, property rights to biological resources could be defined as coterminous with land ownership, and only a private contract with a host country landowner would be required for foreign prospecting organizations to obtain legal access to biological resources. At the other extreme is full nationalization of biochemical information and genetic resources, with national government authorization required for all biochemical prospecting activity. I argue below that a combination of private property rights, national government oversight, and shared compensation is the most effective means of promoting beneficial biochemical prospecting activity.

Defining who has the right to sell access to biological resources for commercial research and development raises the question of to what degree these ownership rights and the ability to exchange them in market transactions should extend to intellectual property derived from biological resources. Some commentators believe that developing-country enforcement of intellectual property rights will inhibit access and use of new technologies and will only ensure that developed countries obtain most of the benefit from biochemical prospecting activities (Shiva 1993). Lax enforcement of intellectual property rights during the early stages of U.S. and Japanese industrial development is often cited as justification for this argument. There is no doubt that free access to existing technologies has its benefits, but the broader costs of eschewing intellectual property rights are often ignored. Advocates of strong intellectual property rights in developing countries argue that a legal and regulatory environment that promotes free access to new innovations will merely foster an entrepreneurial sector that copies from others, yielding only short-term economic returns (Sherwood 1992; Clemente 1988; Haagsma 1988). Sherwood's (1990) research in Latin America provides some empirical support for this hypothesis. He recounts several instances where Latin American researchers have developed new drugs and biotechnologies that have been patented and are under development in the U.S. and Europe but have not been developed in their country of origin because of weak intellectual property protection. Sherwood's surveys of Latin American business managers, corporate research scientists, and venture capitalists also indicate that weak, ineffectual property rights are inhibiting investment in domestic research and development.

An additional argument for strong intellectual property protection in developing countries is based on the implications for technology transfer and foreign direct investment. Foreign pharmaceutical companies and other prospecting organizations are unlikely to engage in significant technology transfer, training, and technical assistance in a country that does not enforce intellectual property rights. Mansfield's (1992) survey of the degree to which intellectual property rights in developing countries affect licensing and direct investment decisions by U.S. firms indicates that the chemical and pharmaceutical industries place the greatest importance on these factors. On average, over 60 percent of chemical and pharmaceutical industry managers indicated that intellectual property protection was too weak to permit licensing their newest or most effective technology in the 13 developed countries targeted in the survey. All of the chemical and pharmaceutical firms that responded to Mansfield's survey indicated that the strength of intellectual property rights had a strong effect on direct investment decisions involving research and development facilities.

If a country is seeking to promote sustainable development of its biological resources, its focus must be on developing a domestic industrial sector capable of deriving economic profits from the chemical and genetic diversity of its biota. Obtaining technology developed elsewhere is essential, but even this may require strong intellectual property protection. In the long run, sustainable development of biological resources will require independent, innovative activity in the host country, which will require appropriate legal protection of intellectual property.

Market Research and Oversight

A critical factor affecting the host country's ability to integrate biochemical prospecting programs into its land-use and economic development plans is the lack of information on such key parameters as the market value of biological samples, the cost of collecting large quantities of samples, and the quantity and quality of the host country's stock of biological resources. At present, no international institution is responsible for monitoring or compiling data on biochemical prospecting activities. In many transactions, such basic information as a description of the samples or extracts, the quantity supplied, and the negotiated compensation are kept secret by both buyers and sellers. Moreover, suppliers of biological samples include third-party collectors, such as botanical societies and academic institutions, that have other motivations besides financial returns for collecting specimens of exotic or previously undiscovered species. These suppliers are often not particularly interested in monitoring the costs of collection and comparing these costs with the price received for samples.

Given the formative, decentralized, and often secretive nature of the biochemical prospecting market, the host country may be able to obtain significant benefits from any information it can obtain about the market value or expected collection costs and other characteristics of its biological resources. For example, developing a network of contacts among potential buyers of biological samples can provide important information on the prices that could be obtained for various quantities of biological extracts with specific characteristics. Sampling programs intended to estimate species diversity within particular ecosystems or more comprehensive efforts (such as the one currently under way in Costa Rica) to inventory and catalogue all species within the country can also provide essential information for resource management.

Although definitive quantification will not usually be possible, some estimate of the benefits of obtaining improved information on market values, species diversity, or collection costs can be developed by comparing the expected value of decisions that would be made on the basis of currently available information with the expected benefits that might be realized if more accurate information were available.[17] In some cases, the value of information may be a significant part of the benefits that the host country obtains from its first few biochemical prospecting efforts. To ensure professional management and long-range planning while maintaining the flexibility to respond to changes in technology and market conditions, it may be appropriate for the government to delegate responsibility for the host country's biochemical prospecting activities to an independent public-sector organization. Whatever the administrative arrangements, it is likely to be advantageous for the host country to develop the means for regulating, monitoring, and reviewing any market transactions involving the country's biological resources.

One inexpensive means for the host country to begin to gather information on its biological resources and their market value would be to require all researchers or collectors to obtain collection permits indicating the types of species to be collected, the purpose of the collection effort, the buyer(s) of any samples collected, and the terms of the sale (Janzen et al. 1993). As part of the permit system, the host government might also require the parties involved to file periodic reports on collection costs and research results. The host government should also be represented in, or at least have the opportunity to review the results of, any negotiations involving the sale of domestic biological material to a foreign organization. This would help to ensure that competing host country suppliers are not undercutting each other on price. Government participation in all contract negotiations related to biochemical prospecting endeavors could also help to ensure that competing host country suppliers are not unnecessarily creating a buyer's market. In addition, the host country would be better positioned to utilize information and expertise gained from previous transactions to increase the benefits derived from future biochemical prospecting efforts.

While a centralized permitting and contract review process could provide significant benefits to the host country, it is important that the process be handled with a minimum of delay and according to consistent and appropriate criteria that are clearly understood by all parties. If the process is too time-consuming or capricious, prospecting organizations will seek opportunities in other countries where biological samples can be obtained more rapidly and with greater certainty. Indeed, host countries should consider implementing streamlined permitting and contract review procedures while providing a broad array of logistical support services, including within-country travel arrangements, field equipment, interpreters, ecologically knowledgeable guides, and collection and delivery of samples.

A more aggressive approach to controlling the market for biochemical resources would be for host countries to develop alliances or cartels, with the aim of managing supplies and coordinating contract negotiations. However, the number of potential source countries is quite large, and many currently have very little control over the export of their biological resources. As a result, it would be very difficult to enforce supply quotas or contract guidelines. In addition, even if an effective supply cartel were organized, host countries would need to be very cautious about increasing prices to a degree that would cause a rapid shift toward alternative sources of novel chemical compounds, such as synthesized molecules or bioengineered variations of commonly available biological material.

As an intermediate step toward supply management, a host country might seek to exchange information and to coordinate biochemical marketing, research, and development efforts with a few neighboring countries that provide habitat for many of the same organisms. For organisms that are found in more than one country in the region, agreements might be established to share biochemical prospecting benefits as a means of forestalling cutthroat supply competition. Countries that are party to these agreements would be required to establish certain controls over transactions involving their biological resources.[18]

Strategic Planning for Research, Development, and Technology Transfer

Developing countries argued for strong technology transfer requirements as part of the Convention on Biological Diversity, which was signed in Rio de Janeiro in 1992, and most recent biochemical prospecting efforts include provisions for technology transfer and technical training by the prospecting organization

(UNEP 1992). The Merck/INBio agreement includes funding for INBio to purchase equipment for extract preparation, testing, and chemical isolation. INBio also receives the benefit of sending members of its technical staff and collaborating Costa Rican scientists for extended training at Merck's U.S. headquarters. Similar arrangements are included in separate agreements between Pfizer and Glaxo and collaborating institutions in the People's Republic of China. The International Cooperative Biodiversity Group Program, which is being funded by NIH, the National Science Foundation, and the Agency for International Development, includes a wide range of technical assistance and training of host country personnel. The NCI's material transfer agreement also includes provisions for training and technical assistance.

Presumably, the primary objective of developing countries in seeking access to biochemical technology and technical assistance is to advance their own biochemical R&D capabilities. As outlined below, there are several good economic arguments for pursuing this objective. Nevertheless, biochemical technology transfer and technical assistance do not automatically translate into economic prosperity. Before negotiating technology transfer, technical assistance, or training programs as part of a biochemical prospecting contract, the host country should develop a strategic plan for technology development that is tailored to the country's needs and capabilities and responsive to market opportunities.

To obtain significant benefits and create conservation incentives in the emerging biochemical prospecting market, countries will have to find or create a market niche that they can at least partially monopolize. By developing and marketing their unique resources, countries would no longer be competing directly against each other in the sale of a generic commodity, such as now occurs in the production of bananas, sugar cane, and copper ore. Rather, they would become monopolistic competitors negotiating unique contracts with biochemical prospecting firms whose needs correspond with the specific resources each country has to offer. In this situation, countries seeking to supply biological material and related technical resources would have greater opportunity to negotiate compensation arrangements that yield an economic profit.

Megadiversity countries could seek to establish themselves as biological supermarkets providing prospecting organizations with access to a vast array of biological samples. Countries with sizable indigenous populations or well-developed systems of medicinal plant use could draw upon their culturally based intellectual resources. Countries with a high percentage of locally endemic species could seek to exploit these unique biological resources. Some countries with low labor costs could initially seek to provide low-cost and relatively high-quality collection and extraction services.

While some brokers of biological material offer samples and extracts for sale with little value added, there are indications that the market for biological resources is already evolving toward monopolistic competition. INBio, in its projects with Merck and Bristol-Myers Squibb, has been focusing on the use of insects as sources of new drug leads. It has also begun efforts to utilize ecological information as a means of increasing success rates in its biochemical prospecting efforts. There is no doubt that Costa Rica is also benefiting from a combination of political stability, an impressive protected area system, and long-standing ties to research institutions in the United States and other highly developed countries. China has negotiated biochemical prospecting contracts with both Glaxo and Pfizer that draw upon the extensive use of medicinal plants in traditional Chinese medicine. The International Cooperative Biodiversity Group (ICBG) project in Surinam has emphasized the use of ethnobotanical information, while the ICBG project involving researchers from Argentina, Chile, and Mexico is focusing on arid land plants from these three countries.

A first step toward developing a domestic biochemical research and development program would be for the host country to increase the quantity, quality, and accessibility of biological and ethnobiological information. Given the opportunities that the host country has for marketing its biological material to numerous prospecting organizations, there would seem to be a clear incentive for countries to develop specialized knowledge of the pharmacological or other commercial potential of their flora and fauna. For example, if the host country were able to collect biological resource information that leads to improved success rates in biochemical R&D programs, prospecting organizations should be willing to pay higher prices for samples identified through the use of this information. Unfortunately, a price premium may only materialize after reports that a prospecting organization has isolated promising compounds from species identified through the host country's biological research efforts. To provide a tool for monitoring and marketing its ethnobiological or ecological research programs, the host country could contract for independent chemical screening tests of extracts from species identified with the use of this information.

Using ecological or ethnobiological information to identify promising species could be considered a form of prescreening. The next logical step would be for the host country to develop the capability to perform one or more subsequent phases of the biochemical R&D process. While the models developed in Chapter 2 demonstrate that the expected value of a biochemical compound increases as it proceeds through the R&D process, this does not necessarily mean that biologically rich countries can increase the net benefits they receive by selling screened compounds as opposed to unprocessed biological material. Even if the host country develops the capability to screen biological extracts and to isolate promising compounds, the costs of screening thousands of extracts to find one promising lead significantly reduces the net benefits the host country will ultimately receive for each compound that shows promising test results. Only if it can perform certain R&D functions more efficiently than prospecting organizations's or third-party contractors will the host country be assured of increasing the net benefits it receives as a result of its biochemical R&D efforts.

Although it would take many years for most developing countries to be able to directly compete at all levels with large, technically advanced pharmaceutical companies and other biochemical prospecting organizations from Europe, the United States, or Japan, a host country may be able to identify a niche in which it could compete in the short term. Given relatively low wage rates, as well as some training and technical assistance with standardized procedures for extract preparation, screening, and chemical isolation, developing countries with good infrastructure and a moderate level of technical development might be able to quickly develop a cost advantage in the initial phases of natural product research. Even countries or organizations that are at a relatively low level of technical development could begin to move beyond merely supplying biological samples by employing simple and inexpensive prescreens such as the potato disc and brine shrimp bioassays to identify particularly promising extracts. Anderson and colleagues (1991) report that these simple bench-top assays are highly accurate in detecting known antitumor compounds.

The host country can reduce the risks involved in supporting biochemical research and development by obtaining advance orders for extracts or isolated compounds with certain characteristics. Nevertheless, before providing significant levels of compensation, pharmaceutical companies will want to conduct their own evaluations of extracts or isolated compounds identified by host countries as particularly promising. Through the use of a system of progress payments, as described in Chapter 4, host countries could still negotiate significant compensation for these extracts or compounds, contingent on their successful evaluation by interested pharmaceutical companies.

By developing strategic partnerships or contractual arrangements with companies capable of completing subsequent phases of the natural product R&D process and marketing any resulting products, host countries may be able to develop a critical mass of entrepreneurial and technical skills needed for continued development of biochemical industries. In many cases, nonproprietary technology transfer and training can be provided by the prospecting organization at relatively low cost as part of the prospecting effort. To justify increased technology transfer and technical assistance, host country institutions might consider entering into full partnerships with foreign prospecting organizations, or at least providing some combination of loans and equity investment to the prospecting program. Under this arrangement, the host country would be accepting a greater share of the financial risks of the project in exchange for access to proprietary technology, information, and training. This approach is being promoted by Andes Pharmaceuticals, which is developing a network of suppliers and research institutions in Latin America with an equity stake in the company. Andes has negotiated contracts with collectors and researchers in Colombia and is currently seeking financing to establish pharmaceutical research laboratories in Colombia and the United States (Asebey 1996).

An even more aggressive approach to technology development would be for host country institutions to simply purchase the equipment, licenses, technical services, and training necessary to initiate the country's own biochemical prospecting program. In this arrangement, the host country would retain all profits from the prospecting effort but would also be completely liable for any losses. Once the host country has accepted all or a significant portion of the risks of a prospecting effort, the importance of ensuring that a market exists for any successfully developed products becomes quite clear.

There are also good economic arguments for developing countries to use technology transfer arrangements as a means of developing new pharmaceutical products for their own citizens. Tropical diseases are generally not a major research focus within the pharmaceutical industry simply because many of those who are afflicted by them do not have sufficient resources to provide pharmaceutical firms with an expectation of a reasonable return on their investment. Although the expected revenues of introducing a new drug in the host country may be quite small, the social benefits could be substantial, thereby justifying development of a targeted pharmaceutical R&D program by the host country. The model presented in Chapter 2 could be utilized by the host country to evaluate the expected social benefits of technology transfer in the context of a domestic pharmaceutical R&D program.

Countries with strong ethnomedicinal traditions could also promote the development of a modern natural product research program by introducing incentives for more systematic research and product development efforts into their existing markets for traditional medicines.[19] The basic concept would be to provide either the requirement of formal regulatory approval or the option of authoritative certification for commercially marketed natural product preparations. The exact requirements for regulatory approval or certification would have to be set to provide meaningful information to the public about product efficacy but without being so stringent and expensive as to discourage firms from submitting products for review. If this balance can be struck, it would motivate domestic firms to develop the capacity for natural product screening, clinical trials, and marketing. A requirement for regulatory approval and/or a clear marketing benefit from certification would lead firms to begin to isolate and purify the active ingredients in natural product preparations. Competition would also be expected to spur firms into conducting more broad-based screening programs in an effort to develop new products. Firms would eventually be expected to develop the capacity to synthesize and modify isolated natural products that have been identified in their screening programs.

The Traditional Medicines Program (TRAMED) at the Department of Pharmacology, University of Cape Town, has been promoting an initiative of this sort in South Africa in conjunction with the Medical Research Council, the National Botanical Institute, and the South African Indigenous Plant-Use Forum (Gericke 1994). As part of the TRAMED program, researchers are currently evaluating how to adapt phytomedicinal regulatory regimens employed in other countries for use in South Africa. The Plantas do Nordeste program of the Royal Botanic Gardens at Kew also includes an initiative to screen traditional medicinal plants of the arid northeast region of Brazil and train local urban populations to grow and prepare the most effective remedies (Royal Botanic Gardens 1994).

Auctions and Options

Another proactive strategy that could be used by the host country to manage its biological resources would be to periodically administer auctions of biochemical prospecting rights and/or biological samples. The auctions could involve rights to prospect on public lands or samples supplied from public lands, as well as prospecting rights or samples supplied by private landowners within the country. Of course, host governments would have to determine how to compare the benefits provided by each bid proposal. The analytical framework outlined in Chapter 4 can be used to evaluate a wide range of compensation arrangements. To simplify the analysis, the host government might specify the types of compensation that can be included in each bid, the minimum acceptable compensation, and the minimum acceptable substitution rates between various forms of guaranteed and contingent compensation. The objective would be to reduce the costs of preparing and reviewing bids without restricting bidder creativity to the degree that would prevent consideration of a potentially superior compensation package.

For auctions involving prospecting rights to specific locations, bidders will obviously want to obtain information on the characteristics of these sites. If a narrowly defined set of prospecting rights is to be auctioned, such as the right to collect and test plant samples for potential cardiovascular applications, all bidders are likely to be seeking much the same information about the prospecting location(s). In this situation, it is in the interest of the host country to minimize bidders' site evaluation costs, since these costs will tend to be duplicative and will therefore reduce the amount of the winning bid (Barzel 1982; French and McCormick 1984; Leffler and Rucker 1991). Providing all bidders with reliable information on the size, topography, road network, and other features of the site(s), as well as the results of relevant biological research conducted by reputable third parties, would help to reduce bidders' requirements for independent information. However, if the auction involves broadly defined prospecting rights to one or more complex, biologically rich ecosystems, prospective bidders are likely to be interested in different types of biological material for very different reasons. In this case, site evaluation by bidders will not be completely duplicative and would be expected to increase the amount of the winning bid or bids (Leffler and Rucker 1991; Ramsey 1980).

Another means by which the host country could integrate the potential value of biochemical prospecting into its conservation and development programs would be to sell options to biochemical samples or prospecting rights. A call option for biological samples would give the buyer the right to purchase a specified list of biological samples at a predefined price at some future date or series of dates. Similarly, a call option for unrestricted prospecting rights to a particular location would provide the buyer with the option to collect an unlimited number of samples from these locations, at some future date or series of dates, for a predefined aggregate price. Numerous variations of these options could also be constructed. For example, the host country could sell an option to collect an unlimited number of samples from one or more locations at some future date for a predefined price per sample.

An options market for biochemical resources could provide hedging opportunities for both the host country and prospecting organizations. In addition, analysis of the prices offered for options to biological samples or prospecting rights would provide the host country with important information on the value of its biological resources.

Broadening the Distribution of Benefits

In addition to estimating whether aggregate benefits and costs of a biochemical prospecting endeavor are positive, it is important for the host country to consider the distribution of costs and benefits. This distributional analysis can be critical to the long-term success of the host country's prospecting programs. Economic activities and land-use decisions of local communities and local landowners often have the greatest impact on biodiversity conservation and loss at the prospecting location(s). This is often true even if the prospecting location is a national park or other protected area. Land-use decisions on private lands that border the park, as well as legal or illegal resource extraction activities within the park, can significantly influence its ecology and species composition (Janzen 1986; Lovejoy et al. 1986). By providing local residents, including both landowners and landless workers with an economic stake in protecting the region's biodiversity, it is more likely that potentially valuable species will be preserved for current and future prospecting efforts.

One means of sharing the benefits of biochemical prospecting, which has been adopted by INBio in Costa Rica, is to train local residents to identify and collect biological samples and specimens. INBio has trained a corps of parataxonomists to assist with its ongoing program of inventorying Costa Rica's entire flora and fauna. They are paid a fixed salary and receive basic training in taxonomy, field biology, and the ecology of the regions in which they are collecting samples. More recently, INBio has used funding from the ICBG program to train a group of paraecologists who would use information about the interactions between species to guide biochemical prospecting efforts.

Another rationale for sharing the benefits of prospecting programs is derived from a broad-based conception of intellectual property rights. The basic argument is that if information provided by traditional healers, farmers, or other local residents is used to identify potentially valuable biological materials, then these individuals or their communities should receive a share of the revenues generated from any products derived from these materials (Barton and Christensen 1988; McNeil and McNeil 1989). The critical issue, however, is not whether indigenous or local knowledge providers deserve to be compensated but how much compensation they should receive and how it should be distributed. A prospecting organization may be relying primarily on its own scientific research or it may be utilizing valuable information gathered from local residents. If it is guided by local knowledge to test certain species, it may develop a new product with essentially the same therapeutic or commercial use as the original biological material, or it may discover entirely new uses for the material. In each case, appropriate compensation would differ.

One basis for determining the compensation due to providers of traditional knowledge would be to determine the value added by this knowledge. Unfortunately, once a new product is developed from biological material identified with the help of local knowledge, it is difficult to determine what the net revenues or public benefits from the prospecting endeavor would have been in the absence of this information. Nevertheless, some general compensation guidelines might be developed if the host country and prospecting organization were to compare the costs and success rates of screening programs for ethnobiologically selected samples with the costs and success rates realized using other selection strategies discussed in Chapter 2. The compensation guidelines should also take into account whether the final product had the same basic use as the original material. In addition, since traditional knowledge is, by definition, a social construct, any compensation derived from its use should generally be provided to local communities as opposed to individuals. This is the approach being taken by Shaman Pharmaceuticals, which has established a separate nonprofit organization, The Healing Forest Conservancy, for redistributing part of the revenues derived from ethnobiologically based natural product research back to indigenous communities in the form of local development projects (Moran 1995).

A more ambitious property rights strategy would be to give private landowners a conservation incentive by sharing some portion of the royalties or profits with them if the species from which a new product was developed has been documented to exist on their land. This concept has been proposed on a global scale, but it may be more manageable on a national basis (Vogel 1994; Subramanian 1992). Minimizing fraud in this type of distributed property rights system, particularly for mobile species, would pose formidable administrative problems. Nevertheless, granting all landowners a partial property right for identification, registration, and preservation of species located on their land would provide a direct incentive for private and communal landowners to assist the host government with species inventories and biological conservation programs.

I have argued that central government oversight of or involvement in negotiation of biochemical prospecting contracts can increase host country benefits by minimizing price competition between suppliers within the same country. If the host country is working to develop its own biochemical R&D program and has begun to systematically collect ethnobiological information on its flora and fauna, there are also strong arguments for developing a coherent policy for sharing benefits with local communities. National guidelines for local community compensation acknowledge the value of information provided by indigenous peoples and local residents and provide an incentive for traditional knowledge to be preserved, shared, collected, and analyzed. To the degree that the host government has asserted some control over biochemical prospecting within its borders, a portion of any financial compensation received from prospecting endeavors could be required to be deposited in a national fund for conservation and local sustainable development. Further requirements could also be established for compensation of traditional information used in the prospecting effort. Other project-specific arrangements could be made in excess of these minimum compensation requirements, depending on the nature of the project and the degree of local community involvement.

Chapter 4

Contractual Arrangements
for Allocating Risks and Rewards

INTRODUCTION

A contract is the principal means by which the costs, risks, and rewards of a business venture are allocated between the participating parties. For biochemical prospecting projects, contractual negotiations are likely to focus on the extent and exclusivity of the rights to the biological resources being granted, as well as the form, timing, and amount of financial and in-kind payments. Understanding and, where possible, quantifying the implications of alternative compensation and risk-sharing arrangements can be helpful in negotiating superior terms for biochemical prospecting contracts. Understanding the implications of various contractual arrangements can also be of value to international organizations seeking to promote an equitable and efficient biochemical prospecting market.

EXCLUSIVE PROSPECTING RIGHTS

There are strong reasons for a profit-seeking biochemical prospecting organization to seek exclusive rights to biological resources in contract negotiations. If the prospecting contract does not prevent the supplier from providing biological samples from the same species to other parties during the term of the contract, there is an increased risk that the prospecting organization might not be the first to obtain patents for any compounds developed from the chemicals derived from these species. Since patenting of a new chemical entity normally occurs before clinical trials begin, this additional risk could be modeled as a chance event affecting the outcome of exploratory research. In the baseline analysis presented in Chapter 2, reducing the success rate of the third phase of exploratory research by 20 percent would reduce the after-tax expected net present value of the prospecting effort from $7.3 million to $1.6 million. This simple analysis indicates why a profit-seeking prospecting organization would find it important to obtain exclusive rights to extracts.

Various types and degrees of exclusive rights can be defined for biochemical prospecting endeavors. These include exclusivity in terms of biological material, geographic focus, and prospecting objectives. Merck's contract with INBio is an example of partial exclusivity over a predetermined list of species. The contract prohibits INBio from selling the same extract to another organization for the duration of the contract. The contracts for the ICBG projects contain similar provisions.

Contractual arrangements that prohibit all but one prospecting organization from searching in specified locations provide geographically exclusive prospecting rights. A less comprehensive form of geographic exclusivity might only provide exclusive rights to any samples that the prospecting organization is the first to collect from one or more sites, while still allowing other organizations access to these sites. Geographically exclusive prospecting rights might also restrict what other activities or land uses are permitted in and around the prospecting locations.

For a public research organization such as the National Cancer Institute, exclusive rights of any sort would theoretically be of little value, since their supposed interest is in performing basic research, the results of which are intended to become public information.[1] For a profit-seeking organization, the value of exclusive rights should be a function of the biogeography of the species and/or prospecting locations of interest, as well the prospecting organization's perceptions of the intentions and capabilities of its competition. If the species from which extracts are to be obtained can be found in numerous other countries, then there is little value to the prospecting organization in gaining exclusive rights to these extracts from just one country. Similarly, if the prospecting organization's principal competitors are not emphasizing natural product research, the value of exclusivity is also reduced. Conversely, a high degree of endemism in the species of interest and strong natural product research programs at competing organizations would tend to increase the value of an exclusive contract from the perspective of a for-profit prospecting organization.

In addition to explicitly defining the degree of exclusivity in terms of some combination of species, prospecting locations, and permissible economic activities, the contract should clearly specify the duration of any exclusive rights and whether and how these rights can be extended or renegotiated. Many prospecting contracts provide the prospecting organization with the option of extending its exclusive rights to the extract based upon the results of preliminary screening.

From the perspective of the host country, granting any form of exclusive rights restricts its economic options. The cost of this restriction is a function of the degree of exclusivity, the potential interest in the relevant biological resources from other prospecting organizations, and the value of the prospecting locations for other economic activities. Contractual provisions limiting other prospecting organizations' access to certain species or prospecting locations create opportunity costs for the host country. The less common the biological resources to which access is being restricted are and the greater the demand for these resources is, the greater the opportunity cost to the host country of providing some form of exclusive rights to one prospecting organization.

If the prospecting organization is a public research institute, is supported by international development or conservation funding, or is simply motivated by environmental concern, it may seek to include provisions in the contract that promote conservation at the prospecting location(s). To the degree that these contractual provisions would prohibit other land uses in or around the prospecting locations, this creates an additional opportunity cost of the prospecting effort that should be incorporated into the host country's decision analysis. Not only must the foregone benefits of these other land uses be evaluated, but also the benefits of the prospecting contract must now be estimated without the option to convert the prospecting locations to these other land uses, at least for the duration of the contract.

In theory, it should be possible to define exclusivity quite specifically in terms of species of interest, research objectives, and duration. Under this framework, the host country could grant exclusive rights to test certain species for certain therapeutic objectives for a given time period. Or, the prospecting organization could be granted exclusive rights to obtain any species from a particular geographic area for testing in relation to specific research objectives. The benefit of narrowly defined exclusivity is that the host country can contractually provide the specific rights and safeguards desired by the prospecting organization while retaining the option to negotiate with other organizations that might have a somewhat different interest in the same species or locations.

Enforcement is the principal problem with narrowly defined exclusive rights. The host country would have to incorporate clearly defined research objectives into the prospecting contracts (which would restrict the prospecting organization's options), and the host country would have to demonstrate the ability to monitor and enforce these provisions. It could be quite difficult for a host country to prevent the prospecting organization from collecting unauthorized specimens and even more difficult to prevent unauthorized types of research. However, the risk of negative publicity or even the possibility of losing patent rights for research results related to unauthorized uses of biological material could provide prospecting organizations with strong incentives to abide by the terms of the contract.

If the host country is risk averse, then it is possible that it would be willing to grant exclusive prospecting rights to an interested organization even if the expected monetary value of potential contracts for nonexclusive rights is higher. In general, however, the host country should only be willing to grant exclusive prospecting rights if the expected utility of the exclusive contract is greater than the expected utility associated with the potential combinations of nonexclusive rights that the host country could sell. If V_x is the present value of compensation associated with an exclusive contract to some set of biological resources, $p(V_{nx})$ is the probability of negotiating some combination of nonexclusive contracts to the same resources over the same time period with a total present monetary value of compensation equal to V_{nx}, and the host country's utility function in relation to different levels of monetary compensation from the prospecting contract is defined by U, then the host country should only accept an exclusive contract if the following inequality holds:

$$U(V_x) \geq \int p(V_{nx}) U(V_{nx}) dV_{nx} \qquad (4.1)$$

An important issue to consider jointly with the degree of exclusivity is the prospecting organization's requirements with regard to confidentiality. Without exclusive rights, many prospecting organizations may be unwilling to disclose to the host country the therapeutic objectives of their effort or may seek to prohibit the host country from revealing the identity of the species that are being sampled. Other prospecting organizations might lose interest in certain prospecting locations if they cannot be certain that other prospecting organizations have not obtained samples of the same species. Given this scenario, a nonexclusive—but completely confidential contract—could effectively reduce the value of the host country's biological resources for a certain period of time. If this were the case, it might be more advantageous for the host country to obtain whatever additional compensation it can by explicitly providing the first prospecting organization with a carefully defined set of exclusive prospecting rights.

ALLOCATING FINANCIAL RISKS AND RETURNS

Any prospecting effort entails substantial risk. The magnitude and timing of product revenues or public benefits are uncertain, as are the costs of initial screening and subsequent R&D phases. In any prospecting endeavor involving the collection of large numbers of biological samples from relatively remote locations there is also substantial uncertainty over the cost of collecting these samples. Typically, it is the host country and/or some third-party collector or broker that bears the financial risks associated with collection costs, while the prospecting organization accepts most or all of the risks associated with variability in R&D costs and any resulting revenues or public benefits. However, by explicitly estimating the potential variability in all aspects of costs and benefits—from collection of biological samples to marketing of new products—it may be possible to design risk-spreading arrangements that increase the utility of all affected parties. The principal means of allocating risks and returns between the contracting parties involve the form and timing of compensation for access to biological material.

One of the most common decisions facing the prospecting organization involves the tradeoff between a fixed payment for biological samples and some form of compensation (e.g., royalties) that is contingent on the outcome of the prospecting effort. In comparing fixed and contingent forms of compensation, the first step is defining how each is calculated. The rights and obligations of each party must also be clearly defined. With respect to royalties, it is essential to define whether the royalty will be calculated as a percentage of gross or net revenues and before or after taxes. If royalties are defined simply as a percentage of before-tax gross revenues, then the expected present value of the royalty payment can be calculated by multiplying the royalty percentage by *PVEGR,* as defined in Equation 2.5, by the royalty percentage. If royalties are defined as net of taxes, marketing, and production costs, then the expected present value of the royalty payment can be computed as a percentage of *PVENR,* as defined in Equation 2.6.

A profit-sharing agreement is simply a royalty calculated as a percentage of after-tax revenues net of R&D, production, and administrative costs. The models developed in this chapter can be used to compare these different compensation arrangements. Calculation of the expected present value of profit shares requires an additional step of determining how revenues and expenditures that occur at different points in time will be treated. The most straightforward approach is to deduct all expenditures involved in producing the product from the resulting revenues regardless of their time of occurrence. This approach would not be advantageous from the point of view of the prospecting organization because the majority of expenditures, in the form of R&D costs, occur well before any revenues are received. To account for the time value of money, it would be necessary to discount all costs and revenues to the start of the prospecting effort using the prospecting organization's opportunity cost of capital. This is essentially the expected net present value of the prospecting effort. Therefore, the expected payments from a profit-sharing agreement that took account of the time value of money can be computed as a percentage of the *ENPV* of the prospecting effort as defined in Equation 2.9. An equivalent result can be obtained by increasing the value of prior expenditures at a rate equivalent to the costs of capital and then deducting these compounded costs from current revenues.

For the baseline analysis, involving 15,000 compounds and ten different therapeutic indicators in the primary screening phase, the expected present value of a 1 percent royalty (defined as a percentage of gross revenues) is approximately $2.9 million, or slightly more than $195 per extract. The expected present value of a promise to pay 1 percent of new drug revenues, net of marketing and manufacturing costs, would be approximately $0.8 million, or $53 per extract, in the baseline analysis. In comparison, each 1 percent of new drug revenues net of marketing, manufacturing, and R&D costs, inclusive of the opportunity cost of capital, has an expected present value in the baseline analysis of only $73,000, or slightly less than $5 per extract.

It is instructive to consider the maximum royalty rate that a prospecting organization would be willing to pay given the assumptions of the baseline analysis. If no delivery payments or other forms of compensation are made, the expected return on the prospecting effort would fall below the prospecting organization's opportunity cost of capital if the royalty paid on gross revenues exceeds 2.5 percent. If royalties are calculated on revenues net of marketing and manufacturing cost, then the maximum royalty rate that the prospecting organization could be expected to pay would be approximately 9.2 percent.

VARIATION IN RETURNS FROM ROYALTY AND PROFIT-SHARING AGREEMENTS

If the prospecting organization is risk averse, it will be concerned not only with the expected value of its payments under different compensation arrangements but also with the potential variance in its profits (or benefits) net of these payments. Sebenius and Stan (1982) have shown that for a risk-averse firm, profit sharing will

always be preferable to a fixed payment where the expected value of
the profit share and if the fixed payment are equal. However, Sebenius and Stan also show that, contrary to popular wisdom, royalties
are not necessarily preferable to a fixed fee of equal expected value
and profit sharing is not necessarily preferable to royalty payments.
In both cases, the relative merits of each form of compensation for
the risk-averse firm depend on the covariance between the revenues
and costs of the project. By utilizing correlated probability distributions instead of point estimates for the cost and revenue parameters
of the model presented in Chapter 2, it is possible to estimate probability distributions of expected net present value under various compensation arrangements. These distributions, together with a utility
function or other ranking system that consistently reflected the prospecting organization's risk preferences, could be used to compare the
merits of alternative compensation arrangements.

If the host government maintains a diversified portfolio of assets
and investment projects and if the financial risks of this portfolio are
equivalent to only a small fraction of per capita income, there are
strong arguments as to why the government should act as a risk-neutral investor in negotiating biochemical prospecting contracts (Arrow
and Lind 1970). A counterargument to the Arrow and Lind framework is that use of a risk-neutral investment rate in public project
evaluation would draw resources away from more productive private
investments. In addition, regardless of the theoretical arguments for
the use of a risk-neutral discount rate in evaluating public projects,
there is a tendency for public bureaucracies to be quite risk averse in
practice. This may be the result of a political process that punishes
public officials for failures more than it rewards them for successes.
Whatever the reason, if the host country, or the individuals represent-
ing it, are risk averse, then the comparison of guaranteed versus
contingent compensation should also take into account the potential
variation of royalties, profit shares, or other form of contingent compensation included in the proposed prospecting contract.

For a proposed contract involving royalties, it is the joint probability distribution of the number of successful products emerging
from the prospecting effort and the potential revenues from each
new product that must be determined to understand the potential
variation in returns to the prospecting organization and host coun-

try. If a utility function, $U(x)$, can be defined for each party with respect to the net monetary returns of the prospecting contract, then contract negotiations regarding contingent versus guaranteed payments can be expressed as a maximization problem. From the combinations of guaranteed and contingent compensation that are acceptable to the prospecting organization, the host country is seeking to find the combination that will maximize its utility. Using the binomial distribution to compute the probability of developing a given number of new products, the maximization problem for the choice between guaranteed compensation versus royalties can be defined formally as[2]

$$
\underset{\pi, PVGC}{Max} \sum_{i=0}^{N} \int_{0}^{\infty} (\frac{N!}{A_i!(N-A_i)!})(S^{A_i}(1-S)^{N-A_i} p(PVGR) U\{A_i p PVGR + PVGP\} dPVGR
$$

$$
s.t. [PVGP, \pi] \in Z \text{ and}
$$

$$
\text{mean of } PVGR = MN \prod_{i=1}^{n} S_i \sum_{t=Y}^{Y+T} R_i(1+\delta)^{-t} \tag{4.2}
$$

where π is the royalty rate, $PVGC$ is the present (monetary) value of any guaranteed compensation from the contract, $PVGR$ is the present value of average gross revenues from each new product,[3] $p(PVGR)$ is the probability of a particular value of gross revenues, N is the number of extracts to be screened, M is the number of distinct product objectives that are being screened for in the prospecting program, n is the number of phases in the R&D process, Y is the expected duration of the R&D process, T is the expected life of a new product, δ is the risk-neutral discount rate, A is the number of successful products resulting from the prospecting effort, S is the anticipated overall success rate for each extract, and Z is the set of all combinations of guaranteed payments and royalty rates that are acceptable to the prospecting organization.

Equation 4.2 is, in fact, a simplification of the problem, since the overall success probability is also a random variable for which a probability distribution should be utilized instead of a single parameter. However, given the problems associated with defining utility functions for the prospecting organization and host country, even greater simplification may be justified. One approach would be to calculate a frequency distribution for a few potential ranges of monetary compensation associated with each contractual alternative under review. These frequency distributions could then be used by the participants in the negotiations in reaching a qualitative assessment of which combination of guaranteed and contingent compensation is preferred.

The construction of a frequency distribution for the compensation associated with a particular contract proposal might begin with the use of a truncated Poisson distribution to calculate an approximate probability of developing A new products, as shown below:[4]

$$p(A) = e^{-NS}(NS)^A/A! \qquad (4.3)$$

Probabilities could be calculated for values of A that summed to 95 percent or 99 percent probability. The remaining probability would be assigned to the successful development of one more new product. For example, if S, the overall probability of success for each extract tested, is .00005 and N, the number of extracts tested, is 25,000, the probability of developing more than four new products from the prospecting effort is less than 1 percent.

The second step in the calculation would be to calculate simple probability distributions for ranges of total revenue derived from A new products. If product revenues are assumed to be normally distributed, the density function of the average revenue of A new products would also be normally distributed with its mean equal to the expected revenue of a single new product and its standard deviation defined by the standard error of the expected mean, given that A new products are developed.[5] What this means is that as more products are developed from a particular prospecting effort, the expected probability distribution of the average revenues of these products collapses toward the expected mean revenue of a single product.

Each potential number of new products and its associated probability would then be multiplied by the probability distribution of average new product revenues associated with that value of A. These values and associated joint probabilities could then be condensed into a summary probability distribution of potential royalties. Any guaranteed compensation included in the contract should be added to each range to generate an overall probability distribution for the total compensation of the proposed contract. This procedure is summarized in Table 4.1 for a hypothetical prospecting contract, and the resulting probability distribution is presented in Figure 4.1.

PROFIT SHARING

One theoretical benefit of profit sharing relative to other forms of contingent compensation is that it should not affect the decisions of the prospecting organization regarding whether to continue testing samples. Given a compensation arrangement based solely on profit sharing, a risk-neutral prospecting organization would be expected to continue to test samples as long as the present value of expected revenues (benefits) net of R&D and all other costs is positive. However, if the prospecting organization must pay a fixed fee for each sample or has agreed to pay royalties on any new products, and expected net revenues are positive but less than the fixed payment or expected royalties, the prospecting organization would not be expected to continue with the prospecting effort.

To develop a probability distribution for contingent compensation under profit sharing, it is necessary to estimate the distribution of R&D and other expenses as well as the potential number of new products and their projected revenues. As might be expected, there is some evidence that the success of the R&D effort will be partially dependent on the level of R&D expenditures (Jensen 1987). Consequently, it may be necessary to estimate the joint probability distributions for the number of new products (A), the present value of individual product revenues ($PVNR$), and the present value of R&D expenditures ($PVTC$).[6] Given these joint distributions, the utility maximization problem for combinations of profit sharing and guaranteed compensation can be defined as

$$\underset{\pi,PVGP}{Max} \int_0^\infty \int_0^\infty \sum_{i=0}^{N} (p(A_i \setminus PVTC) f(PVNR, PVTC)$$

$$U\{[\pi A_i PVNR - PVTC] + PVGP\} dPVTC \, dPVNR$$

(4.4)

where π is now the percentage of profits received by the host country, *PVGP* is the present value of guaranteed payments received by the

TABLE 4.1. Calculation of Probability Distribution of Royalty Payments

Number of biological samples (N)	15,000	Royalty rate on gross revenues	1.5%
Overall probability of success (S)	0.00005	Exp. pres. value of gross revenues of a new drug	$250,000,000
Expected # of new products (N * S)	0.75	Std. dev. of pres. val. of gross revenues	$100,000,000

Distribution of Pres. Value of Gross Revenue from a New Drug (PVGR)		Est. Prob. of Occurrence	# of New Drugs (A)	Est. Prob. of of Occurrence*
$0	- $50,000,000	0.02	0	0.472
$50,000,000	- $150,000,000	0.14	1	0.354
$150,000,000	- $250,000,000	0.34	2	0.133
$250,000,000	- $350,000,000	0.34	3	0.033
$350,000,000	- $450,000,000	0.14	4	0.006
$450,000,000	- $500,000,000		5	0.001

*Estimated from poisson dist. given N and S.

Ranges of Pres. Value of Royalty Payments		Est. Freq. of Occurrence*
$0	- $0	0.47
$0	- $2,400,000	0.06
$2,400,000	- $4,800,000	0.26
$4,800,000	- $7,200,000	0.10
$7,200,000	- $9,600,000	0.05
$9,600,000	- $12,000,000	0.03
$12,000,000	- $16,800,000	0.02
	Total	1.00

*Derived from joint prob. dist. of mean of PVGR given A

FIGURE 4.1 Probability Distribution of Present Value of Royalty Payments from Hypothetical Prospecting Project Defined in Table 4.1

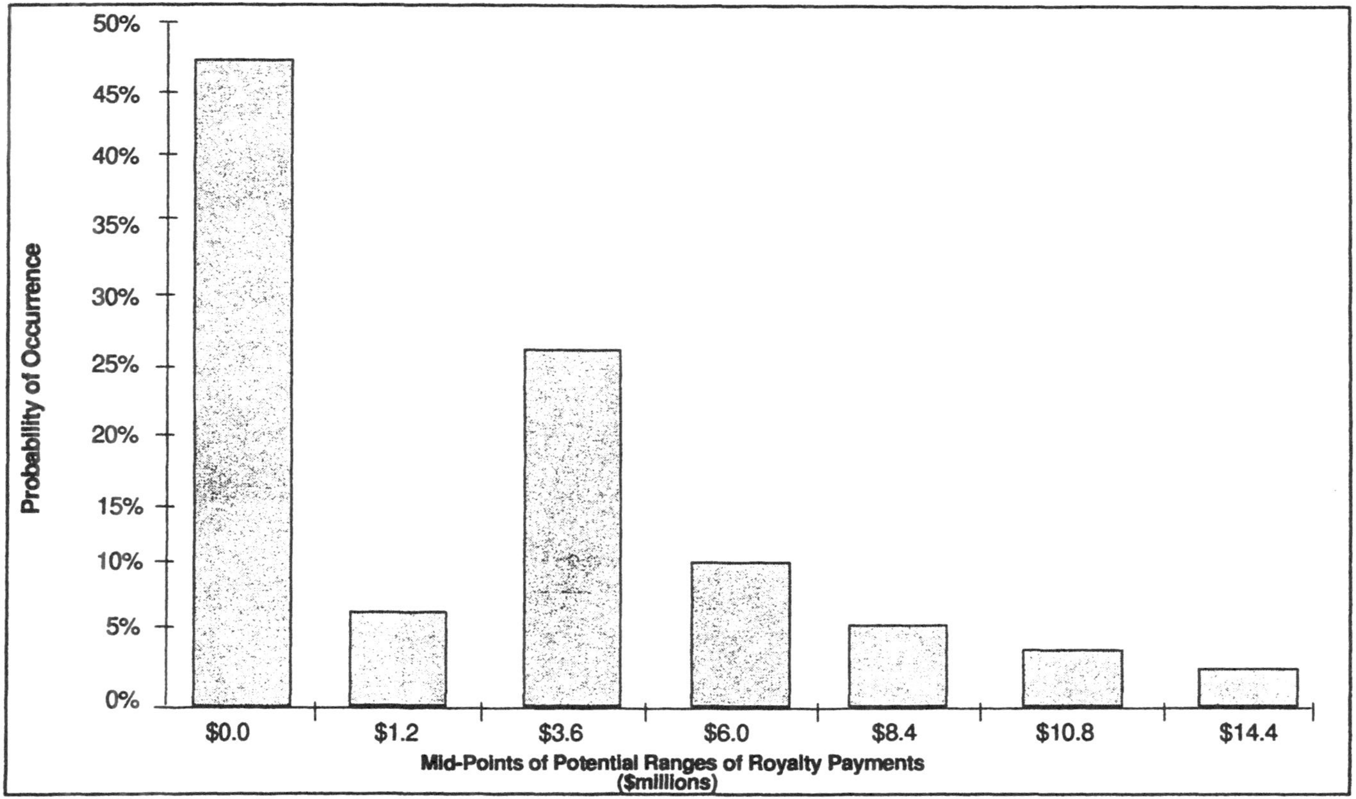

host country, $f(PVNR, PVTC)$ is the joint probability density function of $PVNR$ and $PVTC$, and

$$p(A_i|PVTC) = (\frac{N!}{A_i!(N-A_i)!})(S|PVTC)^{A_i}(1-S|PVTC)^{N-A_i} \quad (4.4a)$$

which is the conditional probability of developing A_i new products, given R&D expenditures equal to $PVTC$.[7]

The potential variability of R&D costs is a function of the probability distribution for the success rate of each R&D phase and uncertainty in the cost of testing an extract or compound at each stage. Variability in R&D success rates also affects the expected profit share as a result of changes in the probability of developing a given number of new products. The prospecting organization or host country could deal with these complications by treating some of the less critical variables as fixed parameters and generating an approximate frequency distribution as described above for royalty agreements. Another alternative is to explicitly establish joint probability distributions for all relevant parameters and then use a computer simulation program to generate an approximate frequency distribution for the proposed prospecting contract. The results of a Monte Carlo simulation of a hypothetical prospecting endeavor with a profit-sharing arrangement are summarized in Figures 4.2 and 4.3, with supporting detail provided in Appendix A.

The calculation of expected utility summarized by Equations 4.2 and 4.4, as well as the simplified frequency distribution analysis described above, assumes that the host country has certain knowledge of the number of extracts (N) that will be tested by the prospecting organization. In fact, there are incentives for the prospecting organization to retain the right to stop accepting extracts, even if the agreed upon quantity has not yet been delivered. Without this right of refusal, the prospecting organization would not be able to benefit fully from information contained in the early results of the primary and secondary screening phases. Conversely, if the prospecting organization must complete the prospecting effort once begun or make significant advance payments, the value of obtaining sample information prior to agreeing to a large-scale prospecting program is increased. In this case, the prospecting organization may want to negotiate a contract that permits testing of a relatively small

FIGURE 4.2. Simulated Distribution of Returns to Prospecting Organization with 15% Profit Share to Host Country*

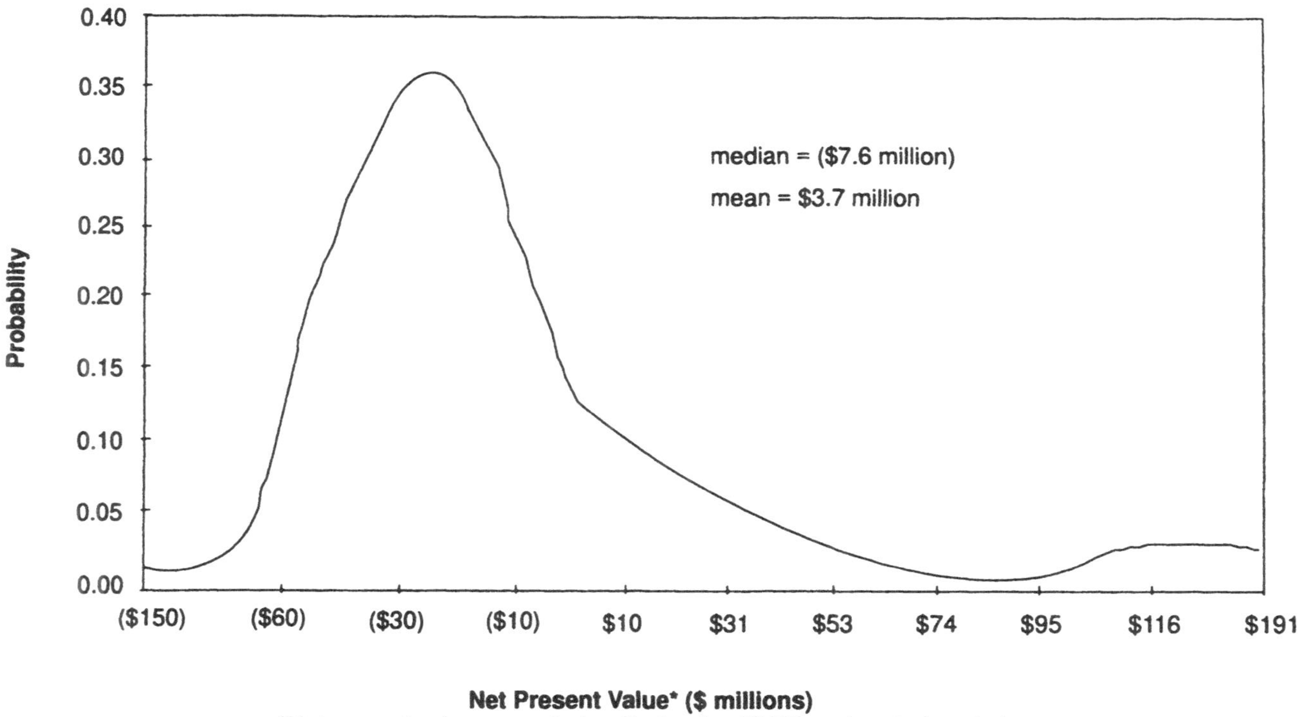

median = ($7.6 million)

mean = $3.7 million

Net Present Value* ($ millions)

*Net present value computed on the basis of 8.5% real cost of capital.

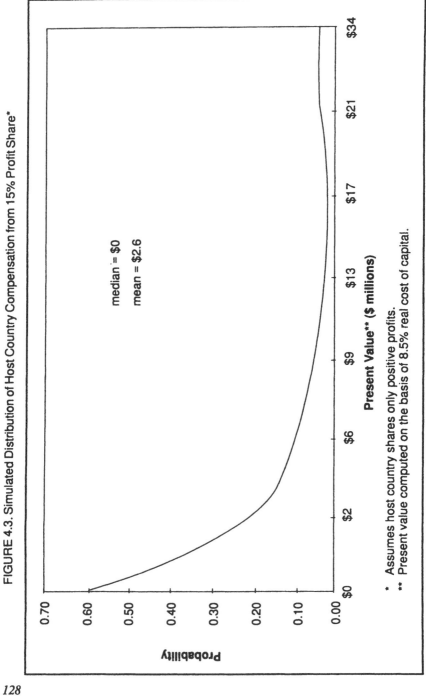

FIGURE 4.3. Simulated Distribution of Host Country Compensation from 15% Profit Share*

median = $0

mean = $2.6

Probability

Present Value** ($ millions)

* Assumes host country shares only positive profits.
** Present value computed on the basis of 8.5% real cost of capital.

sample of extracts with an option to buy a larger quantity if the sample results are encouraging.

There will be even greater uncertainty over the number of samples likely to be tested if the prospecting contract provides for unlimited prospecting rights as opposed to the delivery of a specific number of samples. To determine the expected number of samples to be collected in this situation, the host country must develop estimates of the prospecting organization's marginal cost of collecting each sample. The marginal collection cost function defined in Chapter 3 could be incorporated into the expected utility calculations of Equations 4.2 and 4.4, or the simulation described previously.

If R&D expenditures and new product revenues are not strongly positively correlated, profit-sharing arrangements would result in a shift in risk from the prospecting organization to the host country relative to a fixed-rate royalty agreement (Sebenius and Stan 1982). However, a serious problem with profit sharing from the perspective of the host government is the difficulty of verifying the R&D and other expenses associated with products generated from the prospecting endeavor. The prospecting organization could be required to keep a separate accounting of all expenses and revenues associated with the prospecting contract. However, the difficulty of allocating overhead and other shared expenses opens the door to excessive cost allocation on the part of the prospecting organization. Accounting difficulties such as these have caused problems for profit-sharing agreements for oil and mineral leases (United Nations 1983).

OTHER ARRANGEMENTS FOR ALLOCATING FINANCIAL RISKS AND RETURNS

A common feature of many oil and mineral development contracts is a sliding-scale royalty based upon the level of production or sales. In the case of prospecting contracts, the sliding scale might be based upon the number of successful products generated from the prospecting contract or more directly on the level of annual gross revenues derived from products of the prospecting program. Linking the royalty percentage to the level of sales minimizes risk for the prospecting organization and increases it for the host country relative to a fixed-rate royalty agreement. Equation 4.2, or the simplified frequency distribution described above, can easily be modified to incorporate sliding scale royalties by allowing the royalty rate, π, to vary with the present value of gross revenues.

Another form of sliding-scale contingent compensation that is often included in biochemical prospecting contracts is a royalty rate based upon the level of chemical modification made to the original natural compound. The rationale for modification-based royalties is to compensate the prospecting organization more fairly for its R&D contributions. If the biologically derived compound must be significantly modified, the ratio of original "biological capital" to intellectual property is lower, and an argument can be made that less compensation is due to the supplier of the biological material. The problem with this form of compensation is the inherent difficulty in defining the degree of chemical modification. In addition, it creates incentives for the prospecting organization to pursue unnecessary modification simply to reduce royalties. These problems might be reduced—but not entirely eliminated—if a competent and impartial third party is named in the contract to determine the degree and importance of the chemical modification.

A more direct economic rationale for modification-based royalties is that the prospecting organization is likely to have spent greater sums on R&D for these modified natural products and, all other things being equal, will therefore earn lower profits. Since the degree of therapeutically valuable chemical modification is likely to be correlated with R&D expenditures, profit sharing and variable royalties based on chemical modification may have similar risk-spreading characteristics. But since R&D and other product development expenditures are probably a better measure of the level of effort expended and risk assumed by the prospecting organization, profit sharing is arguably a more equitable means of allocating risks and rewards.

A hybrid solution that achieves some of the same risk-spreading and efficiency objectives as profit sharing but minimizes the accounting difficulties is a system of adjustable royalties based upon the level of new product revenues net of certain easily determined and verifiable expenses. Deductible expenses might include the market value of any other form of taxes paid or compensation provided to the host country or the predefined value of technology transfer and training of host country personnel. Directly related R&D or product development expenditures that take place within the host country might also be deducted from revenues prior to computing the royalty. This would provide added incentives for the prospecting organization to locate a greater share of its project-specific operations within the host country, thereby promoting technology transfer and local employment opportunities.

Progress payments are a form of financial compensation that can be used to strike a balance between the host country's desire to obtain guaranteed benefits early in the prospecting effort and the prospecting organization's desire to make payments only if the project is successful.[8] A set of progress payments might be structured in relation to successful completion of various aspects of the R&D process. The expected present value of a set of progress payments tied to the successful completion of various R&D phases can be computed from the following equation:

$$EPV_{pp} = \sum_{j=1}^{n} \prod_{i=1}^{j} s_i P_j / (1 + \delta)^{T_j} \qquad (4.5)$$

where s_i is the probability of success in phase i, P_j is the progress payment to be made after successful completion of phase j, δ is the annual discount rate, and T_j is the expected time necessary to complete all R&D phases up to and including phase j.

As an example, suppose that the prospecting organization agreed to make a $10,000 payment to the host country for each novel chemical compound discovered in the prospecting effort that is deemed worthy of further research and development. In addition, a $100,000 payment would be made for each compound that advances to the first phase of clinical trials, a $250,000 payment for each compound that advances to the second phase of clinical trials, and a $500,000 payment for each compound that advances to the third phase of clinical trials. For the baseline analysis outlined in Chapter 2, the expected present value of this compensation arrangement would be $2 million, or approximately $136 per extract.

The potential variation in compensation that would result from a progress payment agreement could be explored using the techniques described above for royalty agreements and profit shares. In general, the host country would be expected to prefer progress payments to either royalties or profit sharing, since the probability distribution of progress payments would have a lower variance than either royalty or profit-sharing arrangements of equal expected present value.[9] Prospecting organizations would be expected to prefer progress payments to guaranteed payments but would generally prefer to pay royalties rather than make progress payments as long as there is not a high covariance between product revenues and R&D costs.

SUPPLY GUARANTEES AND RENEGOTIATION CLAUSES

Collection agreements usually require provision of a relatively small amount of biological material for initial testing (NCI 1994; Laird 1993, p. 108). Therefore, a major concern of any prospecting organization is the ability to obtain additional supplies of a sample from which a valuable lead has been developed. Various types of arrangements could be included in the initial contract. At a minimum, the prospecting organization will want to ensure that collection procedures of the host country or its agents include proper identification and geographic information for all samples. The prospecting organization will usually also seek to include in the contract some form of guarantee regarding additional supplies sufficient for further R&D on extracts that show promise in preliminary screening.

Resupply clauses could range from a simple statement indicating that compensation for future supplies will be negotiated once a promising lead has been identified to a full guarantee that the host country will provide future supplies at a previously agreed level of compensation. If a rare species cannot easily be domesticated and compensation arrangements can be renegotiated after preliminary screening has identified a useful lead, then the host government would appear to have improved its bargaining position. The analysis presented in Chapter 2 indicates that the expected value of a compound increases after successful completion of each R&D phase. Assuming synthesis of the active compound is not practical in the short term, the host country would then be in a position to press for compensation approaching the full expected value of the compound to the prospecting organization at that stage of the R&D

process. For these species, the prospecting organization would naturally prefer to lock in a compensation rate prior to initial screening.

For species that can be easily domesticated or whose geographic range includes several countries, the effects of deferring negotiation of a compensation rate are a bit more ambiguous. If other countries or private sources were willing to supply extracts from the organism for little more than the cost of collection, there would be little advantage to deferring negotiation of compensation until a valuable lead had been discovered. In general, potential differences in market conditions for locally endemic versus geographically common species can lead to very different negotiating strategies for the host country, which provides further justification for the host country to increase its knowledge of its biological resources.

A MARKET FOR ROYALTY RIGHTS AND PROFIT SHARES

To the degree that stockholders in a private pharmaceutical company hold a diversified set of investments, they should not be concerned with the total risk of the prospecting project, but with how the returns of the project vary in relation to other investments in their portfolio. Similarly, the host government should consider the correlation between the net benefits of the prospecting project and other economic activities in the country. Since the net benefits of the prospecting project may bear little relationship to the profits earned by the sale of other commodities or manufactured goods produced by the host country, the risks of the prospecting project may be nearly eliminated in relation to the total portfolio of the host country.[10]

Nevertheless, other financial and political considerations may cause managers of the prospecting organization and officials of host country organizations to accept a lower expected rate of return in exchange for a reduction in the potential variability of those returns. Consequently, I shall assume that the host country is to accept less than $1 of guaranteed compensation in exchange for a $1 reduction in the expected present value of contingent compensation. Conversely, I shall assume that the prospecting organization is willing to pay more than $1 of expected contingent compensation in exchange for a $1 reduction in guaranteed compensation (i.e., its marginal rate of substitution between contingent and guaranteed compensation is greater than one).

In the absence of a market in which the host country could sell its royalty or profit-sharing rights, the host country should therefore negotiate a compensation arrangement where its marginal rate of substitution between contingent and guaranteed compensation is equal to that of the prospecting organization, as shown in Figure 4.4. However, given the existence of a thirdparty investor who is less risk averse than the prospecting organization or given an impersonal market through which the host government could sell its contingent compensation rights, the optimal contract arrangements from the perspective of the host government would include a higher proportion of contingent compensation. The host government could then increase its welfare by selling some portion of its contingent compensation rights to this less risk-averse investor, as illustrated in

FIGURE 4.4. Pareto Optimal Combination of Guaranteed and Contingent Compensation

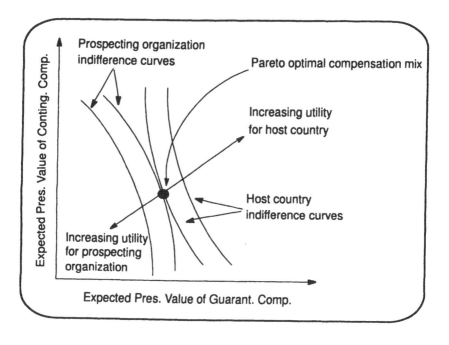

Figure 4.5. It is important to note that if the opportunity costs of the prospecting contract to the host country exceed the value of the total compensation offered by the prospecting organization, then the presence of a market for contingent compensation rights would not only increase the benefits received by the host country but would also be necessary for the prospecting endeavor to proceed at all. I will return to this point in the context of international policy options discussed in Chapter 5.

FIGURE 4.5. Pareto Optimal Compensation Mix Given Market for Contingent Compensation Rights

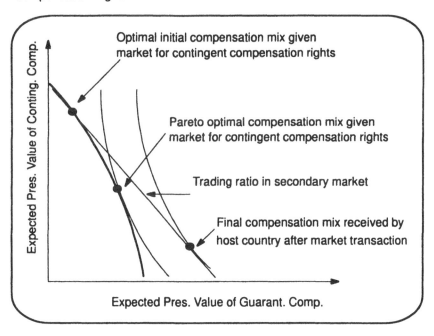

TECHNOLOGY TRANSFER, TRAINING, AND TECHNICAL ASSISTANCE

The principal reason why the host country might seek to obtain technology and training as part of a biochemical prospecting contract is to increase the benefits it can derive from its biological resources. Of course, biochemical technology and training are not valuable goods in and of themselves. They become valuable only in the context of a coherent research and technology development program on the part of host country institutions involved in the biochemical prospecting program. This might include the creation of R&D programs focusing on diseases of concern to the host country, or it might focus on increasing the net benefits derived from the sale of biological resources by performing certain aspects of the R&D process in-country.

Determining the value of proprietary technology or technical assistance to the host country requires an assessment of the degree to which the technology will increase revenues or public benefits obtained by the host country from future biochemical prospecting endeavors. Using the model presented in Chapter 2, the host country could estimate the net benefits of its biochemical R&D efforts with and without access to the proprietary technology as a means of determining the technology's value. For nonproprietary and widely available technology and technical assistance, the market price for these goods and services establishes an upper limit on their value to the host country.

The prospecting organization may be able to provide both proprietary and nonproprietary technology and technical assistance relatively inexpensively if this is done as part of an ongoing biochemical prospecting project. There is very little additional cost in providing significant training to host country scientists by allowing them to participate in field and laboratory activities. The prospecting organization may even benefit from the increased technical capabilities of the host country organizations, since this might reduce the cost or increase the probabilities of success for both the current and any future joint prospecting endeavors.

The potential benefits of technology transfer and technical assistance to the host country, combined with the relatively low cost of providing equipment and training on the part of the prospecting organization, can make these nonmonetary aspects of the prospecting project a pivotal element in negotiations. For example, the host country may be able to increase the benefits it receives from the prospecting contract by trading a somewhat lower level of financial compensation for a significantly greater degree of technology transfer and technical assistance. Similar arguments can be made for trade-offs involving technology transfer and exclusivity of prospecting rights, resupply guarantees, acknowledgment of intellectual property rights, and other issues of concern to the prospecting organization.

INTELLECTUAL PROPERTY RIGHTS

The biochemical prospecting contract should delineate how inventorship is defined and assign rights and responsibilities for patents. Acknowledgment of developing country researchers and indigenous groups as inventors or coinventors in patent filings can have important psychological benefits. Attribution of inventorship can also provide the host country, indigenous group, or individual researcher with prestige that brings benefits in the form of future biochemical prospecting investments. Still, the critical issue is how the revenues and other benefits of a discovery are divided among the parties. Indeed, given the significant expense involved in maintaining and enforcing patents, it is often in the best interests of the source country to assign its intellectual property rights to the prospecting organization in exchange for an appropriate share of any resulting revenues.

SUMMARY AND CONCLUSIONS

I have addressed the question of contractual arrangements from the perspective of two or more parties seeking to maximize the benefits received by the investors or citizens they represent. Within the parameters established by national and international laws and protocols, the parties to the contract are faced with the problem of finding combinations of financial compensation, technology transfer, and property rights that will maximize their own welfare while still being acceptable to the other party. The prospecting organization is seeking guaranteed and exclusive rights to a diverse supply of biological resources as inexpensively as possible. The host country is seeking a high level of compensation for its biological resources and enhancement of its development options. Both parties are likely to be concerned with both the average value of the benefits they can expect to receive under the contract as well as the potential variation in these benefits. By understanding and, where possible, quantifying the potential costs and benefits of various contractual options, participants in the contract negotiations can identify superior arrangements that will increase value for both parties.

Chapter 5

International Policy Implications

POLITICAL ECONOMY
OF BIOLOGICAL RESOURCES

Biologists have come to think of genetic material as a form of encoded information (Alberts et al. 1989). In this context, the value of any component of biodiversity is dependent on the degree to which this biological information has been interpreted. As knowledge about a species increases, its genetic and biochemical information is gradually deciphered and becomes available for productive use. But even a newly discovered species or an ecosystem thought to harbor many unknown species has value as a possible source of new discoveries.[1]

Over time, some forms of commercially valuable biological information can become economically disassociated from the species that was the original source of this information. For example, individual genes or biochemical compounds can often be mass produced using biotechnological methods or chemical synthesis, with little or no need to obtain new material from the source species. Subsequent modifications of the gene or the compound can further remove it from its biological origins. Consequently, as scientific research and technological development proceeds, the potential information that is inherent in biodiversity is translated into intellectual property that is no longer dependent on the biological material from which it was derived.

Information, including biochemical information, is essentially a nonrival commodity (Arrow 1984, p. 142; Aylward and Barbier 1992; Subramanian 1992). Utilization by one individual does not prevent its use by others. If a particular biologically derived compound or gene is used by one firm to create a new drug, there is no *physical* impediment to reproduction and use of the same compound or genetic material, even though this might affect the economic returns to the originating firm.

Historically, biological resources have been treated as being nonexclusionary as well as nonrival. Although countries or individual property owners could theoretically prevent others from obtaining biological material located within their borders, in practice this has proved very difficult (Kloppenburg 1988). Many biological resources grow and reproduce in the wild over broad geographic ranges that often cross international political boundaries. Limiting access to this terrain and preventing unauthorized transport of biological specimens can be prohibitively expensive. Moreover, as techniques for ex-situ conservation, domestication, chemical synthesis, and genetic engineering have advanced, the quantity of biological material needed to secure access to important commercial discoveries has continued to decline. Intended or unintended transport of a few seeds or samples can, in a short time, result in a major redistribution of sources of supply for biochemical resources.

The nonrival and nonexclusionary characteristics of biochemical resources, together with the important role that research plays in revealing their value, have provided intellectual support for the treatment of biological resources as the "common heritage of humanity." If use by one individual does not limit use by others and if increases in knowledge about a species create new wealth, then why not make biological material freely available to all for continued research and knowledge generation? Once the difficulty of limiting access to biological resources is acknowledged, the relative benefits of open access appear even greater. In 1983, the concept of the common heritage of mankind was formally incorporated by the Food and Agriculture Organization (FAO) into the International Undertaking on Plant Genetic Resources.[2] The common heritage concept continues to form the basis of the current international system of gene banks and crop research centers.

Unfortunately, this line of reasoning ignores the detrimental effects of open access with regard to the conservation and sustainable utilization of biological resources. The detrimental incentives created by uncontrolled open access are widely recognized in relation to natural resources such as fisheries, rangelands, and the atmosphere. Indeed, most environmental law and natural resource management efforts are focused on how to restrict access to common property resources through the use of pricing systems or the creation of new forms of property rights.

Open access has also been rejected as a basis for managing intellectual resources. Patent systems and other forms of intellectual property rights are based on the assumption that if the benefits of new inventions cannot be at least partially appropriated, potential generators of new information and innovations have little incentive to engage in the effort. With regard to information associated with biological resources, concern over the incentives provided for innovation and knowledge generation has led the International Union for the Protection of New Varieties of Plants, which includes most developed countries, to adopt a system of plant breeders rights (PBR) that is akin to patent protection. In addition, patents are routinely granted by developed countries for discoveries related to the particular uses of naturally occurring compounds, their synthetic variants, and processes for generating them (Bent et al. 1987).

While open access has until recently been the universally accepted norm for raw biological material, intellectual property rights have been in existence for some time for commercially valuable information related to these resources. This two-tiered system creates a set of perverse incentives for those most responsible for safeguarding the world's biodiversity. Without an opportunity to receive compensation for the information inherent in biodiversity, there is a reduced incentive for individual property owners or nations to preserve these resources. Granted, some incentive exists for countries to preserve their biological diversity until they can perform research and development that would allow them to appropriate the benefits of this information themselves. But such a forward-looking posture is difficult to maintain if a country's current economic opportunities are largely limited to more traditional exploitation of its natural resources.

Several researchers have suggested that the creation of new forms of national, communal, and individual property rights pertaining to wild plants and animals would result in greater conservation and more efficient utilization (Sedjo 1988; Subramanian 1992; Aylward and Barbier 1992; Vogel 1994). Even without the benefit of universally recognized property rights there have been several recent examples of biochemical prospecting endeavors where the prospecting organization has agreed to compensate the host country for access to biological resources. Merck, Glaxo, Pfizer, Smith-Kline, Bristol-Myers, Syntex, Shaman Pharmaceuticals, and the National Cancer Institute are all presently involved in biochemical prospecting efforts that involve compensating the host country for access to biological material (Reid et al. 1993; Pollock 1992; Grifo 1996; NCI 1994; Armond 1994). Although definitive international recognition of property rights to wild biological material would provide a more secure foundation for this emerging market, it would not automatically result in efficient incentives for conservation and sustainable development of biodiversity.

THE BIODIVERSITY CONVENTION

One way of understanding the Convention on Biological Diversity (hereafter referred to as the Biodiversity Convention, or simply the convention) prepared for the 1992 United Nations Conference on Environment and Development (UNCED) is to regard it as the first hotly debated step away from the historical open-access approach to biological resources toward a more highly managed system of property rights. While ethical concerns regarding the intrinsic value of biodiversity were also an important motivation for many of the participants in the negotiations over the convention, the focus of the convention is on establishing sovereign rights over biological resources, developing mechanisms for their sustainable use, and ensuring an equitable distribution of the resulting benefits (UNEP 1992).

The general objectives of the convention, as defined in Article 1, include the conservation of biological diversity, sustainable use of its components, and the fair and equitable sharing of the benefits resulting from the utilization of genetic resources.[3] A long list of specific measures for achieving these objectives is outlined in the convention. Parties to the convention are expected to

• develop national biodiversity protection plans and programs for sustainable use;

- inventory and monitor components of biological diversity that are threatened, endangered, or of economic, cultural, or scientific value;
- establish a system of protected areas with appropriate guidelines for their selection and management;
- establish and maintain facilities for ex-situ conservation;
- establish programs for scientific research and technical training related to identification, conservation, and sustainable use of biological diversity; and
- integrate consideration of conservation and sustainable use of biological resources into national decision making.

While the preamble to the convention outlines the arguments for preserving biodiversity, it also states that "economic and social development and poverty eradication are the first and overriding priorities of developing countries" and that "special provision is required to meet the [conservation and sustainable development] needs of developing countries, including the provision of new and additional financial resources and appropriate access to relevant technologies." In general, the convention acknowledges that international assistance will have to be provided to developing countries to pursue biodiversity protection efforts that do not provide tangible net benefits to the host country.

The convention also acknowledges the rights of countries to obtain compensation for access to their genetic resources, including transfer of relevant technologies and equitable sharing of research results and other benefits. The ambiguity of the convention on the intellectual property rights and compensation arrangements that should apply to transactions involving genetic resources reflects not only compromises between parties to the negotiations but also the transitional state of legal and economic thinking on these matters.

In comparison with other international environmental treaties, the ratification process for the Biodiversity Convention was unusually rapid. After ratification by more than 30 countries, the convention formally went into effect less than 18 months after its signing at the Earth Summit in Rio de Janeiro. Still, many of the provisions of the convention are quite vague, potentially contradictory, and liberally sprinkled with phrases that essentially leave countries to decide for themselves what constitutes compliance (e.g., "to the maximum reasonable extent"). Moreover, while the convention explicitly states that developing country compliance will be dependent on external financial assistance, the funding sources for the conservation and sustainable development measures outlined in the convention have not yet been determined. Article 20 of the convention simply states that "developed country parties shall provide new and additional financial resources to enable developing country parties to meet the agreed full incremental costs to them of implementing measures that fulfill the obligations of this Convention." However, the principal contributor to multinational assistance programs has generally been the United States, which has signed but not ratified the convention.

The convention that was signed in Rio is therefore only a framework that will require the development of specific protocols and funding mechanisms for effective implementation. Nevertheless, one advantage that the Biodiversity Convention enjoys relative to other international environmental agreements is the potential to draw upon private-sector investments and market forces as a principal means of achieving its objectives. Before reviewing the policy options available at the international level for promoting a biochemical prospecting market, it may be useful to examine some of the reasons for government involvement in this market from the perspective of economic theory.

POTENTIAL IMPEDIMENTS TO AN EFFICIENT BIOCHEMICAL PROSPECTING MARKET

The potential supply of biological samples is quite large and potentially renewable. Approximately 1.7 million species have been described by science, and estimates of the total number of species range from 5 million to more than 50 million (Hammond 1992, p. 19; May 1990). Moreover, since different parts of the same species may have very different chemical characteristics, the potential supply of chemically distinct biological samples is substantially greater than the number of species. In addition, specimens from a particular species may be tested with more than one technology, for more than one commercial objective, or by more than one firm. Even a species that has been thoroughly screened for all potential uses may again become the focus of biochemical R&D due to scientific and technological developments.

Although there is very little information available on the demand side of the biochemical prospecting market, one recent survey of major pharmaceutical companies and research institutes identified screening capacity in excess of 50,000 samples per year (Reid et al. 1993, pp. 8–13). However, this study includes information from only a few companies and public research institutes. In addition, many of the organizations sampled did not provide complete information on their screening programs, and the study generally did not distinguish between screening capacity and actual number of samples tested. Even assuming that ongoing natural product screening programs completely investigate the commercial potential of 200,000 distinct species a year, it would take nearly a decade to thoroughly evaluate all species currently known to exist. Continued progress in identifying new species and in developing more sensitive screening technologies could allow the *potential* supply of biological samples to satisfy demand for several more decades.

Given the publicity and policy attention that biochemical prospecting has received, there is likely to be increasing competition between suppliers of biological resources. Countries such as Mexico, Colombia, Indonesia, South Africa, and China, to name a few, are actively seeking ways to benefit from the emerging biochemical prospecting market. From one perspective, it is encouraging that countries are beginning to take notice of the potential value of biological resources. Nevertheless, there is reason to believe that competition between sources of supply could keep the price of randomly collected biological samples from rising much above the average cost of collection for the foreseeable future. Unless source countries can generate and supply specialized information or valuable services in addition to biological material, they will find themselves competing in a commodity market with very low profit margins.

One practical difficulty that countries seeking to enter the biochemical prospecting market must contend with is the pricing problem associated with joint production. Even if a country wanted to recover its full costs of biodiversity protection plus some pure rental income for access to enjoyment of this biodiversity, it must still struggle with how to estimate and allocate costs and benefits among a wide range of uses. Natural ecosystems provide a wide range of goods and services, including watershed protection and other ecosystem services; a site for recreation and ecotourist activities; a source of food, medicines, and building materials for local residents; and a set of psychic benefits that economists refer to as existence value. Market prices do not exist for most of these goods and services. Moreover, public officials rarely have accurate information on the maintenance and opportunity costs of national parks, biological reserves, and other publicly owned protected areas. If some public and private landowners are willing to sell biological samples for little more than the variable cost of collection, it makes it difficult for others to bargain for a higher price, thereby reducing the incentive for public officials or private landowners to devote additional land and other resources to conservation efforts.

The problem of joint production and underpricing of biological samples might not be of particular concern if species extinction were reversible. Unfortunately, once a decision has been made to convert a biologically rich natural area to another use, future opportunities for biological prospecting in that ecosystem will have been severely reduced no matter how high the price of biological samples might rise in the future. This simple observation underlies the concept of quasi-option value discussed in Chapter 3. The long-term adjustment mechanisms between supply and demand in the market for biological samples are not the same as those for bananas or computer chips. Once potential sources of biological samples have been eliminated through extinction, these species cannot be resurrected, biotechnological progress notwithstanding.

The economic problems posed by the irreversibility of extinction are only exacerbated by substantial time lags in biochemical research and development. As indicated in Chapter 1, it takes in excess of 10 years—and often as much as 20 years—to develop a new drug and obtain regulatory approval to market it. Even if substantial royalties are promised for any new products developed from biological samples obtained from the host country, by the time any royalty payments materialize, habitat conversion and species extinction may have advanced substantially.

For the moment, however, suppose that all private and public landowners are well-informed about the biodiversity that exists on their land, are attempting to recover the full maintenance and opportunity costs of protecting natural ecosystems, and are aware of the potential royalties and other forms of contingent compensation they could obtain by providing access to biological material. In addition, these landowners have used the techniques discussed in Chapter 4 to determine the present value certainty equivalent of this contingent compensation. Finally, assume public and private landowners are cognizant of trends in biochemical and ecological research that could affect the future value of biological samples (i.e., they are accurately evaluating the quasi-option value of preserving the biodiversity on their land). Even under these unrealistically strong informational and behavioral assumptions, the unregulated decisions of private landowners, prospecting organizations, and nation-states are still not likely to be economically efficient. The decisions of these actors will not incorporate many of the positive externalities associated with biochemical prospecting and conservation of biodiversity.

The social and international benefits of developing new medicines, pesticides, or other products from biological source material are likely to exceed the returns that can be realized by the prospecting organization and the host country, even with very liberal patent protection (Wu 1984; PMA 1992; Mansfield et al. 1977). In addition, the quasi-option value associated with biodiversity preservation will be much greater from a global perspective than from the perspective of the private landowner or host country. There are several reasons for this. First, there are few positive international externalities associated with destruction of a relatively pristine ecosystem for purposes of silvicultural, agricultural, or industrial production.[4] Second, from a global perspective, there are likely to be many more alternatives to this conversion than from the perspective of the host country. Finally, the technologies currently and potentially available at the global level for research and development of biological resources are by definition at least as advanced as those of any country or group of countries. In short, the social value of biochemical prospecting and biodiversity protection can be expected to exceed the private value of these activities, and global benefits are likely to exceed national benefits. Given the positive externalities associated with biochemical prospecting, utility-maximizing decisions of private landowners, corporations, and individual countries would be expected to lead to a lower level of research and development than is optimal from a global perspective.

High transaction costs are another factor that inhibits the efficient operation of an international biochemical prospecting market. At present, it is an expensive and time-consuming endeavor for countries to obtain information on the quantity, quality, distribution, and market value of their biological resources. It is also quite difficult for a prospecting organization to obtain comparative information on biological resources available in several countries. Many potentially beneficial biochemical prospecting opportunities will not be exploited due to difficulties in identifying interested parties, understanding political and institutional risks, and negotiating mutually acceptable contractual arrangements. The transactions that do occur are likely to be suboptimal because buyers and sellers may not be aware of more advantageous opportunities. If biologically rich countries cannot easily obtain accurate information on the market value of biological samples, extracts, and isolated promising compounds, these countries will be unable to make efficient decisions regarding investments in biodiversity conservation and biochemical R&D.

There are a few private firms, such as Biotics Ltd. of Great Britain and Biospecs based in the Netherlands, that have emerged as brokers of biological resources. Many botanical gardens, zoological societies, and oceanographic institutes also provide collection and brokerage services. These organizations provide an important market function that should be supported by international institutions. Nevertheless, just as certain regulations and professional norms have been established for securities and insurance brokers, standard procedures, reporting requirements, and professional guidelines should be developed for brokers of biological material.

The development of an active biochemical prospecting market is also inhibited by a high degree of technological, economic, and political uncertainty, combined with a lack of risk-spreading mechanisms. From the perspective of the prospecting organization, there is a form of option value associated with delaying an irreversible investment until new information becomes available (Pindyck 1991). If a pharmaceutical company is uncertain whether rational drug design and biotechnological developments will make natural product research more valuable or economically obsolete, this uncertainty creates an incentive to delay making a major investment until the underlying trend becomes more obvious. Uncertainty regarding protection of intellectual property rights and international protocols for biochemical prospecting are likely to reinforce a potential prospecting organization's tendency to take a wait-and-see approach.[5] Engaging in a very limited screening program or taking a partial share in a research consortium are less risky means of gathering additional information on the potential benefits of large-scale biological screening. Unfortunately, given the long lead times involved in biochemical R&D, small-scale screening programs may not provide developing countries with much incentive to preserve their biodiversity.

From the perspective of the host country, the potential payoffs from preserving natural ecosystems for biochemical prospecting must be continually evaluated in relation to the economic benefits of competing land uses. However, the degree of risk aversion and the risk-free discount rate associated with economic decisions of a biologically rich—but income-poor—developing country are likely to be much higher than those employed by the international community as a whole. Without improved market mechanisms for transferring risks and translating the long-term, international benefits of biodiversity conservation into more immediate benefits for the host country, developing countries would be expected to preserve less of their biodiversity than would be optimal from a global perspective.

This prediction applies even if developing countries had perfect biogeographic information and excellent knowledge about the market for biochemical prospecting rights. A more realistic set of assumptions would, of course, acknowledge the paucity of information about the world's biological diversity. Informed estimates of the total number of species vary by more than an order of magnitude (May 1990). Knowledge of the geographic distribution of tropical species, including sites of high diversity and/or endemism is largely based on a few surveys of relatively well-known vertebrate and plant species (Bibby, Collar, and Crosby, 1992; Myers 1988 and 1990; WCMC 1992, pp. 581–583). A lack of information regarding the quantity and quality of the host country's biological resources, the low level of compensation currently provided for the potential information inherent in raw biological samples, and uncertainty about technological changes that could affect the future value of resources could be expected to interact with a high discount rate to further reduce the resources developing countries devote to conservation of biodiversity.

INTERNATIONAL POLICY OPTIONS

The emergence of an active biochemical prospecting market would provide an additional means of converting the potential future value of biodiversity into current income for those most responsible for and most affected by the preservation of biologically rich ecosystems. However, as argued above, simply creating a market for biological material may not in itself generate significant conservation incentives or benefits for the host country. Establishing a biochemical prospecting market that will promote conservation of biodiversity and create economic development opportunities will require a coordinated system of protocols, economic incentives, and financing mechanisms. Toward this end, international assistance must be appropriately targeted to complement and promote host country public expenditures, private-sector investments, and community involvement.

The decision models developed in Chapters 2, 3, and 4, together with the economic analysis of this chapter, provide some insight into policy measures that can be used to increase the equity and efficiency of the emerging biochemical prospecting market. These measures can be grouped into four broad categories: market management and intermediation, host country capacity building, international research and development, and financing and risk-spreading arrangements.

Market Management and Intermediation

Article 18 of the Biodiversity Convention includes a requirement for the Conference of the Parties (COP) to establish a clearinghouse to promote technical and scientific cooperation on the sustainable development of biological resources. I believe it would be beneficial for the clearinghouse and other mechanisms for international cooperation to provide a much broader array of information and services. For example, the market value of biological resources is an important input into decisions regarding conservation and land-use planning. Information on innovative financing and contractual arrangements is also of great value to parties seeking to develop biochemical prospecting endeavors. For these reasons, the clearinghouse should seek to maintain and disseminate information on the financial, legal, and institutional aspects of biochemical prospecting activities as well as scientific and technical information.[6]

It would also be quite beneficial if the COP, in conjunction with other international institutions and private organizations, were to support the creation of one or more central exchanges through which host countries, prospecting organizations, and biochemical brokers could indicate their interest in buying and selling specific types and quantities of biological material. The COP, in conjunction with other international institutions, could also assist developing countries in formulating strategic plans for sustainable development of their biological resources while helping to identify organizations that could contribute critical technologies or services in exchange for biochemical prospecting rights. These types of technical assistance and exchange services would serve to reduce transaction costs between buyers and sellers of biological resources and related technologies. Central brokerage and exchange services would also make it easier for the COP to collect, evaluate, and disseminate information on biochemical prospecting activities and their effects on host country conservation efforts and R&D programs.

Lesser and Krattiger (1994) have recommended the creation of a new facilitating organization modeled on the International Service for the Acquisition of Agri-Biotech Applications to promote the exchange of genetic technologies and biological material. Eisner and Beiring (1994) have called for the creation of an international Biotic Exploration Fund, which would provide brokerage services for biochemical prospecting as well as capital for developing-country capacity building. The United Nations Conference on Trade and Development (UNCTAD) is also developing a Biotrade Initiative aimed at facilitating this emerging market through technical assistance and development of protocols (UNCTAD 1995). In addition, several consulting firms and professional organizations, such as the Biodiversity Technology Group (BTG) and the International Organization for Chemists in Development (IOCD), both based in Washington, DC, have begun to provide technical assistance services to countries seeking to develop their biological resources. Through the creation of appropriate protocols, certification, and reporting mechanisms, it may be possible for the COP and international organizations to facilitate the emerging biochemical prospecting market through a network of for-profit and nonprofit entities that provide brokerage, exchange, and technical assistance services.

Developing protocols for biochemical prospecting contracts, including guidelines for financial compensation, technical assistance, technology transfer, and protection of intellectual property rights, would help support this emerging market by reducing uncertainty and transaction costs. However, given the potential complexity and diversity of biochemical prospecting endeavors, international protocols should not be designed to impose standardized forms of compensation and other contractual terms. Imposing—or even promoting—a requirement for an unrealistically high rate of compensation on all bioprospecting contracts would have the effect of stifling legitimate contracts and promoting black market transactions. Rather, the protocols should outline a range of contractual options and provide information that would assist all parties in determining what legal and economic arrangements are appropriate under various circumstances. Indeed, contractual protocols could be most useful as part of a more comprehensive manual or training program for negotiating and managing biochemical prospecting endeavors.

One objective in developing a set of protocols would be to protect host countries from unscrupulous collectors and prospecting organizations. An equally important purpose of protocols and compensation guidelines would be to promote fair competition between host countries by preventing "dumping" of biological samples at prices lower than the fully allocated cost of supply. International guidelines should emphasize that compensation for access to raw biological material be sufficient to recoup not only collection and preparation costs but also an appropriate share of maintenance, enforcement, and opportunity costs associated with protection of the prospecting sites. The manual suggested above might also include methodologies for determining the host country's full cost of biodiversity protection and how these costs could be allocated to individual biochemical prospecting activities.

Compensation guidelines should also emphasize the need for a fair distribution of expected returns in relation to the value added and risks incurred by all parties to the negotiations. Knowledge contributions from local indigenous groups, host country R&D programs, and the prospecting organization's R&D process must all be considered in the analysis. However, value added must be understood as a dynamic concept that varies over time as technologies and market conditions change. Methodologies developed in Chapters 2, 3, and 4 could assist contract negotiators in estimating the risks and expected returns of the prospecting endeavor as well as the value added by each party.

Of course, any effort to promote higher prices for biological samples, if not accompanied by offsetting reductions in other expected costs or risk factors, could eliminate some research efforts that might have led to substantial public benefits. Protocols for financial compensation, technical assistance, and technology transfer should therefore be accompanied by other international initiatives to facilitate biochemical prospecting activities. In addition, guidelines for technology transfer must be developed in relation to requirements for protection of intellectual property rights.

Although some developing countries and international NGOs have been reluctant to support strong IPR provisions in the Biodiversity Convention,[7] it can be expected that those countries that affirmatively protect IPRs will become more attractive sites for private investments in biochemical R&D. Moreover, negotiated technology transfer and technical assistance arrangements are likely to be more generous if the prospecting organization is confident that the host country will not be using proprietary information in a manner that is detrimental to the prospecting organization's competitive position. Technology transfer protocols should therefore seek to promote reciprocity. The prospecting organization should be encouraged to freely share relevant research techniques and results with the host country for use in developing products for its domestic market. Any other uses of proprietary information or technology by the host country should be negotiated in separate licensing agreements. Technology transfer and technical assistance arrangements that are more generous than this baseline should be considered as contributing toward the overall compensation provided by the prospecting organization.

The COP should also consider developing an international certification system for biochemical prospecting activities. Prospecting agreements that complied with all relevant protocols would receive a special certification that could be used in marketing any resulting products. To the degree that receipt of this certification increased sales or investor interest, companies would have an added incentive to undertake biochemical prospecting efforts in accordance with international protocols and to identify the resulting products. Individual countries could provide a powerful incentive for prospecting organizations to seek this certification by making certification a requirement for receiving patent protection on new drugs developed from biological material.

Improving Host Country Information and Technical Capacity

Since preservation of biologically rich ecosystems must often compete with other land uses, one priority for the international community should be to assist countries in improving their knowledge about the quantity, quality (in the terms of rarity or economic potential), and distribution of species that exist within their borders. The need for international financial and technical assistance for species inventories, biogeographic surveys, and ethnobiological studies is widely recognized (Soule and Kohm 1989, pp. 73–74; NRC 1992, pp. 37–40). To obtain maximum benefit from this assistance, it should be targeted toward training host country personnel, such as the corps of parataxonomists employed by INBio in Costa Rica (Soule and Kohm 1989, pp. 79–86; Janzen 1991; Raven and Wilson 1992; Sittenfeld and Gamez 1993).

Improving the quality of a host country's biochemical products and services appears to be the most promising means of increasing host country benefits and providing meaningful incentives for biodiversity conservation. In most cases, biochemical prospecting organizations require that biological samples be supplied with sufficient information to locate additional supplies of samples of interest. Beyond this minimum quality requirement, the ability to supply samples from particular taxonomic groups, preparation of samples into extracts, identification of samples with a greater probability of commercial value, and the performance of preliminary screening are all realistic means by which the host country can increase the value added to its biological products in the near term. Over a longer time horizon, developing the capability to perform chemical isolation and characterization as well as biotechnological processes would permit the host country to capture a greater share of the benefits from biochemical prospecting.

For these technical development initiatives to be most effective, they must be focused on well-defined national needs and international market opportunities (Correa 1991, Juma 1993). In many countries, there is a dire need for strategic planning in relation to the initiation and conduct of biochemical prospecting and related R&D programs. Since biochemical prospecting is a business activity as much as it is a scientific or technical endeavor, training programs are also needed in market research, business planning, intellectual property law, contractual negotiations, and financing mechanisms.

International Research and Development

Given the high fixed costs of technically advanced natural product research programs, it may be appropriate to establish a system of regional centers to perform preliminary screening and subsequent research on the biochemical properties of species common to several countries. There may also be a role for a global system of biochemical prospecting centers with specific research objectives such as the development of new medicines for tropical diseases or the development of biological pesticides. A system of regional and product-oriented research centers would serve a function analogous to the international agricultural research centers managed by the Consultative Group on International Agricultural Research (CGIAR). However, in contrast to the CGIAR's management philosophy, an international system of biochemical research centers should acknowledge sovereign rights to biological resources and develop compensation mechanisms for biological materials and associated intellectual property.

To date, public support for biochemical prospecting efforts has focused on screening of biological samples. The NCI's natural product research effort is essentially a screening program, as is the natural product research component of the NIH/NSF/USAID International Cooperative Biodiversity Group Program. I believe greater attention and additional funding should be given to developing new biochemical screening techniques and biotechnological processes with widespread application to plants, insects, and microorganisms. The catalytic effects of new screening technologies can be observed in the NCI's screening program, which originally used an expensive and time-consuming in-vivo whole-mouse model and then was reinvigorated after the development of an in-vitro assay screening for activity against as many as 60 cancer cell lines. The importance of developing new screening technologies and biotechnological procedures can also be understood through an analogy to fossil fuel exploration and extraction.

At any point in time, total petroleum reserves can be categorized as economic reserves, which include all known deposits that can be profitably extracted given current prices and technologies; known but noneconomic reserves; and potential reserves, which would include additional stocks suspected to exist based on preliminary geological analysis. Extraction of petroleum from existing well fields reduces economic reserves. In contrast, investments in exploration and the development of more efficient petroleum extraction technologies tend to increase economic reserves. The benefits that can be derived from biological resources (i.e., the potential stock of new discoveries) can be analyzed using a similar framework.

Screening biological samples with existing bioassay techniques can be expected to yield a finite number of valuable new products, thereby reducing the stock of untapped economic discoveries. On the other hand, development of more advanced screening technologies, together with continued biodiversity exploration (e.g., species inventories, advances in chemical ecology and biochemistry), would increase economic reserves of new biochemical products. In the long term, the flow of new pharmaceutical products and other material benefits from biodiversity, and the economic incentives for its conservation, will be a function of the rate at which technological and economic advances can discover reserves of biochemical resources and create the techniques with which to "extract" these reserves economically.

Financing and Risk-Spreading Arrangements

International protocols for compensation, technology transfer, and intellectual property rights need to be developed for public as well as privately funded biochemical prospecting activities. For example, the international biochemical research centers proposed above should be encouraged to enter into license agreements and negotiate compensation for any finished products, isolated compounds, or other patentable discoveries for which they are responsible.[8] Compensation might be based on a sliding scale related to the uses that are permitted under the license agreement and the characteristics of the licensee (e.g., nonprofit research institute, multinational corporation, developing-country government agency). Revenues from these agreements should be shared among the research centers themselves and the country or countries that supplied the biological source material. Some of the proceeds from license agreements might also be used to support biodiversity conservation efforts in other countries that are party to the convention and have completed a biodiversity inventory and protection strategy.[9]

The efficiency of transactions involving prospecting organizations and source countries could be increased through the development of a market for royalties rights and other claims to contingent compensation of biochemical prospecting ventures. Figures 4.4 and 4.5 in the previous chapter illustrated the benefits of creating a market through which a risk-averse host country could sell its biochemical prospecting royalty rights to a less risk-averse third party. By allowing the host country to trade uncertain future compensation for guaranteed current compensation, a secondary market for contingent compensation rights could increase the utility the host country receives from biochemical prospecting contracts. Moreover, the opportunity to engage in these transactions expands the set of mutually beneficial compensation arrangements that can be negotiated between the host country and the prospecting organization. As a result, agreements could be reached on some prospecting ventures that would otherwise be left unexploited.

There are several steps that could be taken by the COP or other international institutions (e.g., World Bank organizations) to promote the development of a secondary market for biochemical prospecting compensation rights. A first step might simply involve the expansion of the clearinghouse and brokering functions, described above, to include a service for matching potential buyers and sellers of contingent compensation rights. International institutions might also assist buyers of these rights to monitor the results of relevant research by the prospecting organization.

A more ambitious financing and risk-spreading initiative would involve the creation of an international fund for investments in biochemical prospecting ventures. Although public funding and nongovernment donations could provide seed money for a biochemical prospecting investment fund, the primary objective of the fund should be to leverage and catalyze private-sector investments. The International Finance Corporation (IFC) of the World Bank recently established a venture capital fund to promote sustainable use of biological resources.[10] While the IFC envisions that this fund will ultimately become involved in biochemical prospecting projects, its initial focus has been on ecotourism, sustainable agriculture, and nontimber forest products.[11]

An investment fund focused specifically on biochemical prospecting ventures would offer certain advantages to institutions and individuals seeking to make an investment in this emerging market.[12] First, it could offer specialized expertise necessary to evaluate the biochemical prospecting investments. In addition, it would provide investors with an opportunity to invest in a diversified, and therefore less risky, biochemical prospecting portfolio. The fund could also serve as a conduit for direct investments in biochemical prospecting projects undertaken by private firms, universities, or public research institutes. Any royalties, fees, or other compensation received by the fund would be used to support subsequent biochemical prospecting ventures while providing a return to the fund's investors. As a result, the fund would provide host country institutions and biochemical prospecting organizations with a continuing source of presumably lower cost equity capital.

Another means by which the fund could support the development of an active biochemical prospecting market would be by purchasing biochemical prospecting contingent compensation rights from host countries. As discussed above, these secondary market transactions could expand the level of biochemical prospecting activity while increasing the benefits received by the host country. Direct purchases of contingent compensation rights could be combined with a brokerage function to provide host countries with information on potential buyers of contingent compensation rights before final contract terms have been negotiated with a prospecting organization.

An internationally supported biochemical prospecting fund could also provide financial incentives for host countries to abide by commitments to biodiversity protection. For example, instead of offering immediate payment for contingent compensation rights related to biochemical prospecting ventures, the fund might pay for these rights with a bond that guaranteed annual payments to the host country if it continued to provide appropriate protection to the prospecting location(s). If the host country were a party to the convention, the fund might also require that a certain percentage of these annual payments be devoted to biodiversity conservation efforts specified under the convention.

A biochemical prospecting fund would also have ample incentive and resources to develop effective mechanisms for monitoring the research results of prospecting organizations that are liable to it for royalty or profit-sharing payments. These mechanisms might include reporting requirements, periodic audits, and review of filings for new patents and applications for regulatory review of new drugs or other commercial products.

The development of derivative instruments associated with access to biological resources is another risk-spreading mechanism that deserves international support.[13] A risk-averse host country could increase the benefits it receives from protection of natural areas by selling biochemical prospecting options that provide the buyer with the opportunity to purchase biological material or prospecting rights at a future date. Biochemical prospecting options and other derivative instruments would have the added benefits of providing information on the expected future value of biological resources and a means for investors to hedge their biochemical prospecting risks.

It is important to recognize, however, that one of the essential variables for pricing an option is the price of the underlying asset (Cox and Rubenstein 1985, p. 166), which in this case is the value of the associated biological material or biochemical prospecting rights. Providing increased financial information about transactions involving biochemical prospecting and associated contingent compensation rights would therefore promote the development of a derivative market for biochemical resources. The venture capital fund discussed above might well become an active participant in this derivative market, both as a buyer and as a reseller. This would provide some price information and liquidity to the market while enabling the fund to exercise greater control over the risk-return characteristics of its portfolio.

A derivative market for prospecting rights is unlikely to develop unless investors can be assured that host countries can and will honor their obligations to protect the biological resources on which the derivative instrument has been sold. There is some potential to structure the payments on derivative instruments in ways that would provide financial incentives to the host country to preserve the underlying biological assets. Nevertheless, the involvement of international institutions in providing financial and technical assistance and in monitoring host countries' biodiversity protection efforts could reduce the risks perceived by potential buyers of derivative biochemical prospecting instruments.

SUMMARY AND CONCLUSIONS

In countries with rapidly expanding populations seeking to improve their standard of living, it is difficult to preserve biodiversity if the benefits of doing so are not readily apparent. The increasing private-sector interest in genetic material and other biochemical resources offers an opportunity to translate the long-term value of biodiversity protection into more immediate benefits and conservation incentives. Nevertheless, I have argued that the conditions necessary for an efficient biochemical prospecting market do not presently exist. Property rights to biological resources are not well defined or easily protected. Information about these resources is often insufficient to determine their value or the full costs of supply. Transaction costs are quite high, and risk-spreading mechanisms are not well developed. In addition, the global benefits of biodiversity conservation and biochemical prospecting exceed the benefits that can be appropriated by individual firms or countries. Under these circumstances, biochemical prospecting is unlikely to generate substantial new incentives for biodiversity protection without public support and oversight.

As the market for biochemical resources continues to develop, international institutions should experiment with a wide range of policy measures and organizational arrangements for promoting research, development, and technology transfer. Within this diversity, the focus of international assistance should be on increasing host country scientific, technological, and entrepreneurial expertise while expanding private-sector demand for biochemical resources. There are several mechanisms available for pursuing this objective, including development of international protocols for transactions involving biochemical resources, provision of market information and other intermediation services, publicly supported R&D programs that complement those of the private sector, and support for derivative and secondary markets that expand the opportunities for transferring and spreading risks.

Appendix A

Simulated Distribution
of Returns from Biochemical
Prospecting Opportunity

Summary of Results

Expected Net Present Value

Entire Range is from ($194,514,895) to $326,947,628
After 200 iterations, the Standard Error of the Mean is $3,945,084

Statistics:	Value
Iterations	200
Mean	$4,674,256
Median (approx.)	($7,533,333)
Mode (approx.)	($14,610,324)
Standard Deviation	$55,791,911
Variance	3E+15
Skewness	2.44
Kurtosis	15.44
Coeff. of Variability	11.94
Range Minimum	($194,514,895)
Range Maximum	$326,947,628
Range Width	$521,462,523
Mean Std. Error	$3,945,083.88

Percentile	$ (approx.)
0%	($194,514,895)
10%	($31,123,304)
20%	($20,694,054)
30%	($16,100,217)
40%	($12,136,720)
50%	($7,533,333)

60%	($414,956)
70%	$9,434,892
80%	$23,108,798
90%	$57,525,325
100%	$326,947,628

Average Expected Net Present Value Per Extract
Entire Range is from ($12,968) to $21,797
After 200 iterations, the Standard Error of the Mean is $263

Statistics:	Value
Iterations	200
Mean	$312
Median (approx.)	($502)
Standard Deviation	$3,719
Variance	$13,834,388
Skewness	2.44
Kurtosis	15.44
Coeff. of Variability	11.94
Range Minimum	($12,968)
Range Maximum	$21,797
Mean Std. Error	$263.01

Percentile	$ (approx.)
0%	($12,968)
10%	($2,075)
20%	($1,380)
30%	($1,073)
40%	($809)
50%	($502)
60%	($28)
70%	$629
80%	$1,541
90%	$3,835
100%	$21,797

Mean Values of Parameters Used in Simulation

	Effective Duration (yrs.)	Cond. Prob. of Success Per Trial	Cost per Trial
Primary Screening	0.00	0.005	$100
Secondary Screening	0.10	0.400	$1,000

Isolation & Dereplication	0.50	0.100	$20,000
Synthesis and Modification	1.50	0.500	$250,000
Preclinical Trials	1.00	0.400	$771,317
Clinical Phase I	1.35	0.750	$3,136,980
Clinical Phase II	1.88	0.475	$9,932,790
Clinical Phase III	2.49	0.700	$18,817,470
NDA	3.00	0.900	$1,000,000
Number of Extracts Tested		15,000	
Number of Initial Screens		10	
Chem. Correlation		0.00	
Real Discount Rate		8.50%	
Contrib. Margin		0.40	
Global/U.S. sales		1.90	
Tax Rate		35%	
Pres. Val. of Global Net Rev. from Each New Drug			$80,020,000

Distributions Used for Variable Parameters

Real Discount Rate
Lognormal distribution with parameters:

Mean	8.50%
Standard Dev.	0.75%

Mean value in simulation was 8.51%

Correlated with:	Corr. Coeff.
Drug Revenue Multiplier	0.25
R&D Cost Multiplier	0.25

Chemical Correlation Between Extracts
Beta distribution with parameters:

Alpha	1.00
Beta	19.00
Scale	1.00

Mean value in simulation was 0.05

Success Rate per Trial in Preliminary Screening
Beta distribution with parameters:

Alpha	1.00
Beta	199.00
Scale	1.000

Mean value in simulation was 0.0.05

Success Rate in Modification and Synthesis
Beta distribution with parameters:

Alpha	20.00
Beta	20.00
Scale	1.000

Mean value in simulation was 0.493

Correlated with:	Corr. Coeff.
Expenditures for Mod. & Synthesis	0.50

Preliminary Screening Costs per Trial
Lognormal distribution with parameters:

Mean	$100
Standard Dev.	$25

Mean value in simulation was $100

Expenditures for Synthesis and Modification
Lognormal distribution with parameters:

Mean	$250,000
Standard Dev.	$125,000

Mean value in simulation was $248,488

Correlated with:	Corr. Coeff.
Success rate in Synthesis and Modification	0.50

R&D Cost Multiplier
Value <1 proportionately reduces R&D costs relative to expected value.
Value >1 proportionately increases R&D costs relative to expected value.

Lognormal distribution with parameters:

Mean	1.00
Standard Dev.	0.25

Mean value in simulation was 0.99

Correlated with:	Corr. Coeff.
Distribution of Drug Revenues	0.25
Real Discount Rate	0.25

Drug Revenue Multiplier
Value <1 proportionately reduces drug revenues relative to expected value.
Value >1 proportionately increases drug revenues relative to expected value.

Lognormal distribution with parameters:

Mean	1.00
Standard Dev.	0.50

Mean value in simulation was 1.04

Correlated with:	Corr. Coeff.
Real Discount Rate	0.25
R&D Cost Multiplier	0.25

Secondary Screening Success Rate
Beta distribution with parameters:

Alpha	6.00
Beta	9.00
Scale	1.000

Mean value in simulation was 0.404

Preclinical Trial Success Rate
Beta distribution with parameters:

Alpha	16.00
Beta	24.00
Scale	1.000

Mean value in simulation was 0.397

Clinical Phase 1 Success Rate
Beta distribution with parameters:

Alpha	30.00
Beta	10.00
Scale	1.000

Mean value in simulation was 0.752

Clinical Phase II Success Rate

Beta distribution with parameters:

Alpha	47.50
Beta	52.50
Scale	1.000

Mean value in simulation was 0.479

Clinical Phase III Success Rate

Beta distribution with parameters:

Alpha	28.00
Beta	12.00
Scale	1.000

Mean value in simulation was 0.695

Appendix B

Two-Period, Two-Site, Dynamic Programming Land-Use Planning

Max PVB=for t=1 to $2 \sum [BC_t/(1 + \delta)^{t-1} + BE_t/(1 + \delta)^{t-1} + BP_t/(1 + \delta)^{t-1}]$
     s.t. $0 \leq P_{1,t}, P_{2,t}, C_{2,t} \leq 1$

Benefits of Conversion BC = $\chi_1[A_1,(P_{1,t} - C_{1,t})]^{\alpha 1} + \chi_2[A_2(P_{2,t} - C_{2,t})]^{\alpha 2}$

Benefits of Environmental Services BE = $\lambda_1[A_1(P_{1,t} - C_{1,t})]^{\beta 1} + \lambda_2[A_2(P_{2,t} - C_{2,t})]^{\beta 2}$

Benefits of Prospecting BP = for i=1 to $2 \sum \{\varepsilon_i \gamma_i (A_i)^{Z_i}[1 - r_{iL} R_{i,t}/(R_{i,t} + r_{iL})][v_t - k_i - k_i \ln(v_t/k_i)]\}$

   where $R_{i,t} = [\sum$ for j = 1 to 2 $r_{ij}\varepsilon_j \gamma_j [A_j(P_{j,t} - C_{j,t})]^{Z_j}] - \varepsilon_i \gamma_i [A_i(P_{i,t} - C_{i,t})Z_i \cdot \varepsilon_i \gamma_i (A_i)^{Z_i}$

Parameter Values

A_1	=	10,000	χ_1	=	100	α_I = 0.4	λ_1 = 0.20	r_{12} =	0.20
A_2	=	1,000	χ_2	=	75	α_2 = 0.3	λ_2 = 30	r_{21} =	0.45
γ_1	=	5,000	Z_I	=	0.35	β_i = 0.5	χ_1 = 100	r_{1L} =	0.20
γ_2	=	5,000	Z_2	=	0.35	β_2 = 0.6	χ_2 = 75	r_{2L} =	0.45
ε_1	=	0.5	ε_2	=	0.7				

Initial value of biol. samples v_1 = $300   Years per period = 10
Potential values of stochastic variable $\ominus$ (high) = 2   Annual discount rate $\delta = 0.05$
     (with equal probability) $\ominus$ (low) = 0.5
     Period 2 value of biol. samples $v_2 = v_1 \times 0$

Summary Table of Expected Present Values for Period One Land-Use Choices ($000s)

Degree of Conversion in Period 1		Degree of Preservation at End of Period 1		Conver. Benefits	Env. Serv. Benefits	Biochem. Prosp. Benefits	Total Benefits Period 1	PV Exp. Max. Period 2 Benefits	Total Exp. Benefits Periods 1 & 2
Site 1	Site 2	Site 1	Site 2						
0	0	1	1	0	30,060	6,782	36,842	36,520	73,362
0	0.33	1	0.67	3,299	26,938	6,440	36,677	36,250	72,926
0	0.67	1	0.33	4,079	22,959	5,950	32,988	33,736	66,724
0	1	1	0	4,600	15,443	4,371	24,415	27,769	52,184
0.33	0	0.67	1	19,730	27,257	6,325	53,312	36,533	89,846
0.33	0.33	0.67	0.67	23,028	24,135	5,972	53,135	36,243	89,378
0.33	0.67	0.67	0.33	23,809	20,156	5,463	49,429	33,751	83,180
0.33	1	0.67	0	24,330	12,641	3,799	40,770	27,763	68,533
0.67	0	0.33	1	26,191	23,468	5,674	55,353	36,520	91,873 *
0.67	0.33	0.33	0.67	29,489	20,366	5,302	55,157	36,229	91,387
0.67	0.67	0.33	0.33	30,270	16,387	4,765	51,421	33,736	85,158
0.67	1	0.33	0	30,791	8,872	2,965	42,628	27,684	70,312
1	0	0	1	30,741	14,616	3,670	49,027	31,521	80,548
1	0.33	0	0.67	34,039	11,494	3,190	48,724	31,126	79,849
1	0.67	0	0.33	34,820	7,515	2,490	44,825	28,466	73,291
1	1	0	0	35,341	0	0	35,341	21,696	57,037

Present Value of Benefits for Period Two Land-Use Choices ($000s)

Degree of Preservation at End of Period 1			Conversion During Period 2		Conver.	Env. Serv.	Biochem. Prosp.		Exp. Max.
Site 1	Site 2	⊖	Site 1	Site 2	Benefits	Benefits	Benefits	Total	Benefits
1	1	2	0	0	0	18,454	13,928	32,382	
1	1	2	0	0.33	2,025	16,537	13,297	31,860	
1	1	2	0	0.67	2,504	14,095	12,396	28,995	
1	1	2	0	1	2,824	9,481	9,551	21,856	
1	1	2	0.33	0	12,112	16,734	12,911	41,757	
1	1	2	0.33	0.33	14,137	14,817	12,258	41,212	
1	1	2	0.33	0.67	14,617	12,374	11,321	38,312	
1	1	2	0.33	1	14,936	7,760	8,301	30,998	
1	1	2	0.67	0	16,079	14,420	11,458	41,956*	
1	1	2	0.67	0.33	18,104	12,503	10,767	41,374	
1	1	2	0.67	0.66	18,572	10,143	9,809	38,525	
1	1	2	0.67	1	18,903	5,446	6,479	30,828	
1	1	2	1	0	18,872	8,973	6.870	34,715	
1	1	2	1	0.33	20,897	7,056	5,972	33,925	
1	1	2	1	0.67	21,377	4,614	4,661	30,651	
1	1	2	1	1	21,696	0	0	21,696	
1	1	0.5	0	0	0	18,454	586	19,040	
1	1	0.5	0	0.33	2,025	16,537	544	19,107	
1	1	0.5	0	0.67	2,504	14,095	484	17,083	
1	1	0.5	0	1	2,824	9,481	281	12,586	
1	1	0.5	0.33	0	12,112	16,734	559	29,405	
1	1	0.5	0.33	0.33	14,137	14,817	517	29,471	
1	1	0.5	0.33	0.67	14,617	12,374	455	27,446	
1	1	0.5	0.33	1	14,936	7,760	245	22,942	
1	1	0.5	0.67	0	16,079	14,420	523	31,021	
1	1	0.5	0.67	0.33	18,104	12,503	478	31,085	
1	1	0.5	0.67	0.67	18,583	10,060	414	29,057*	
1	1	0.5	0.67	1	18,903	5,446	191	24,540	
1	1	0.5	1	0	18,872	8,973	428	28,274	
1	1	0.5	1	0.33	20,897	7,056	372	28,326	
1	1	0.5	1	0.67	21,377	4,614	291	26,281	
1	1	0.5	1	1	21,696	0	0	21,696	36,520

Present Value of Benefits for Period Two Land-Use Choices ($000s)

| Degree of Preservation at End of Period 1 | | | Conversion During Period 2 | | Conver. | Env. Serv. | Biochem. Prosp. | | Exp. Max. |
Site 1	Site 2	$\ominus$	Site 1	Site 2	Benefits	Benefits	Benefits	Total	Benefits
1	0.67	2	0	0	2,025	16,537	13,297	31,860	
1	0.67	2	0	0.33	2,493	14,178	12,429	29,100	
1	0.67	2	0	0.67	2,824	9,481	9,551	21,856	
1	0.67	2	0.33	0	14,137	14,817	12,258	41,212	
1	0.67	2	0.33	0.33	14,605	12,458	11,355	38,418	
1	0.67	2	0.33	0.67	14,936	7,760	8,301	30,998	
1	0.67	2	0.66	0	18,007	12,585	10,822	41,414*	
1	0.67	2	0.66	0.33	18,475	10,225	9,866	38,567	
1	0.67	2	0.66	0.67	18,806	5,528	6,547	30,882	
1	0.67	2	1	0	20,897	7,056	5,972	33,925	
1	0.67	2	1	0.33	21,365	4,697	4,710	30,772	
1	0.67	2	1	0.67	21,696	0	0	21,696	
1	0.67	0.5	0	0	2,025	16,537	544	19,107	
1	0.67	0.5	0	0.33	2,493	14,178	486	17,158	
1	0.67	0.5	0	0.67	2,824	9,481	281	12,586	
1	0.67	0.5	0.33	0	14,137	14,817	517	29,471*	
1	0.67	0.5	0.33	0.33	14,605	12,458	457	27,520	
1	0.67	0.5	0.33	0.67	14,936	7,760	245	22,942	
1	0.67	0.5	067	0	18,104	12,503	478	31,085	
1	0.67	0.5	0.67	0.33	18,572	10,143	416	29,131	
1	0.67	0.5	0.67	0.67	18,903	5,446	191	24,540	
1	0.67	0.5	1	0	20,897	7,056	372	28,326	
1	0.67	0.5	1	0.33	21,365	4,697	294	26,356	
1	0.67	0.5	1	0.67	21,696	0	0	21,696	36,250
1	0.33	2	0	0	2,504	14,095	12,396	28,995	
1	0.33	2	0	0.33	2,824	9,481	9,551	21,856	
1	0.33	2	0.33	0	14,617	12,374	11,321	38,312	
1	0.33	2	0.33	0.33	14,936	7,760	8,301	30,998	
1	0.33	2	0.67	0	18,583	10,060	9,772	36,416*	
1	0.33	2	0.67	0.33	18,903	5,446	6,479	30,828	
1	0.33	2	1	0	21,377	4,614	4,661	30,651	
1	0.33	2	1	0.33	21,696	0	0	21,696	

Present Value of Benefits for Period Two Land-Use Choices ($000s)

Degree of Preservation at End of Period 1			Conversion During Period 2		Conver. Benefits	Env. Serv. Benefits	Biochem. Prosp. Benefits	Total	Exp. Max. Benefits
Site 1	Site 2	0	Site 1	Site 2					
1	0.33	0.5	0	0	2,504	14,095	484	17,083	
1	0.33	0.5	0	0.33	2,824	9,481	281	12,586	
1	0.33	0.5	0.33	0	14,617	12,374	455	27,446	
1	0.33	0.5	0.33	0.33	14,936	7,760	245	22,942	
1	0.33	0.5	0.67	0	18,583	10,060	414	29,057*	
1	0.33	0.5	0.67	0.33	18,903	5,446	191	24,540	
1	0.33	0.5	1	0	21,377	4,614	291	26,281	
1	0.33	0.5	1	0.33	21,696	0	0	21,696	33,736
1	0	2	0	0	2,824	9,481	9,551	21,856	
1	0	2	0.33	0	14,936	7,760	8,301	30,998*	
1	0	2	0.67	0	18,903	5,446	6,479	30,828	
1	0	2	1	0	21,696	0	0	21,696	
1	0	0.5	0	0	2,824	9,481	281	12,586	
1	0	0.5	0.33	0	14,936	7,760	245	22,942	
1	0	0.5	0.67	0	18,903	5,446	191	24,540*	
1	0	0.5	1	0	21,696	0	0	21,696	27,769
0.67	1	2	0	0	12,112	16,734	12,911	41,757	
0.67	1	2	0	0.33	14,137	14,817	12,258	41,212	
0.67	1	2	0	0.67	14,617	12,374	11,321	38,312	
0.67	1	2	0	1	14,936	7,760	8,301	30,998	
0.67	1	2	0.33	0	15,982	14,501	11,511	41,995*	
0.67	1	2	0.33	0.33	18,007	12,585	10,822	41,414	
0.67	1	2	0.33	0.67	18,487	10,142	9,830	38,458	
0.67	1	2	0.33	1	18,806	5,528	6,547	30,882	
0.67	1	2	0.67	0	18,872	8,973	6,870	34,715	
0.67	1	2	0.67	0.33	20,897	7,056	5,972	33,925	
0.67	1	2	0.67	0.67	21,377	4,614	4,661	30,651	
0.67	1	2	0.67	1	21,696	0	0	21,696	
0.67	1	0.5	0	0	12,112	16,734	559	29,405	
0.67	1	0.5	0	0.33	14,137	14,817	517	29,471	
0.67	1	0.5	0	0.67	14,617	12,374	455	27,446	
0.67	1	0.5	0	1	14,936	7,760	245	22,942	
0.67	1	0.5	0.33	0	15,982	14,501	524	31,008	
0.67	1	0.5	0.33	0.33	18,007	12,585	480	31,072*	
0.67	1	0.5	0.33	0.67	18,487	10,142	415	29,044	
0.67	1	0.5	0.33	1	18,806	5,528	193	24,528	
0.67	1	0.5	0.67	0	18,872	8,973	428	28,274	
0.67	1	0.5	0.67	0.33	20,897	7,056	372	28,326	

Present Value of Benefits for Period Two Land-Use Choices ($000s)

Degree of Preservation at End of Period 1			Conversion During Period 2		Conver. Benefits	Env. Serv. Benefits	Biochem. Prosp. Benefits	Total	Exp. Max. Benefits
Site 1	Site 2	0	Site 1	Site 2					
0.67	1	0.5	0.67	0.67	21,377	4,614	291	26,281	
0.67	1	0.5	0.67	1	21,696	0	0	21,696	36,533
0.67	0.67	2	0	0	14,137	14,817	12,258	41,212	
0.67	0.67	2	0	0.33	14,605	12,458	11,355	38,418	
0.67	0.67	2	0	0.67	14,936	7,760	8,301	30,998	
0.67	0.67	2	0.33	0	18,007	12,585	10,822	41,414*	
0.67	0.67	2	0.33	0.33	18,475	10,225	9,866	38,567	
0.67	0.67	2	0.33	0.67	18,806	5,528	6,547	30,882	
0.67	0.67	2	0.67	0	20,897	7,056	5,972	33,925	
0.67	0.67	2	0.67	0.33	21,365	4,697	4,710	30,772	
0.67	0.67	2	0.67	0.67	21,696	0	0	21,696	
0.67	0.67	0.5	0	0	14,137	14,817	517	29,471	
0.67	0.67	0.5	0	0.33	14,605	12,458	457	27,520	
0.67	0.67	0.5	0	0.67	14,936	7,760	245	22,942	
0.67	0.67	0.5	0.33	0	18,007	12,585	480	31,072*	
0.67	0.67	0.5	0.33	0.33	18,475	10,225	417	29,118	
0.67	0.67	0.5	0.33	0.67	18,806	5,528	193	24,528	
0.67	0.67	0.5	0.67	0	20,897	7,056	372	28,326	
0.67	0.67	0.5	0.67	0.33	21,365	4,697	294	26,356	
0.67	0.67	0.5	0.67	0.67	21,696	0	0	21,696	36,243
0.67	0.33	2	0	0	14,617	12,374	11,321	38,312	
0.67	0.33	2	0	0.33	14,936	7,760	8,301	30,998	
0.67	0.33	2	0.33	0	18,487	10,142	9,830	38,458*	
0.67	0.33	2	0.33	0.33	18,806	6,528	6,547	30,882	
0.67	0.33	2	0.67	0	21,377	4,614	4,661	30,651	
0.67	0.33	2	0.67	0.33	21,696	0	0	21,696	
0.67	0.33	0.5	0	0	14,617	12,374	455	27,446	
0.67	0.33	0.5	0	0.33	14,936	7,760	245	22,942	
0.67	0.33	0.5	0.33	0	18,487	10,142	415	29,044*	
0.67	0.33	0.5	0.33	0.33	18,806	5,528	193	24,528	
0.67	0.33	0.5	0.67	0	21,377	4,614	291	26,281	
0.67	0.33	0.5	0.67	0.33	21,696	0	0	21,696	33,751

Present Value of Benefits for Period Two Land-Use Choices ($000s)

| Degree of Preservation at End of Period 1 | | | Conversion During Period 2 | | Conver. | Env. Serv. | Biochem. Prosp. | | Exp. Max. |
Site 1	Site 2	0	Site 1	Site 2	Benefits	Benefits	Benefits	Total	Benefits
0.67	0	2	0	0	14,936	7,760	8,301	30,998*	
0.67	0	2	0.33	0	18,806	5,528	6,547	30,882	
0.67	0	2	0.67	0	21,696	0	0	21,696	
0.67	0	0.5	0	0	14,936	7,760	245	22,942	
0.67	0	0.5	0.33	0	18,806	5,528	193	24,528*	
0.67	0	0.5	0.67	0	21,696	0	0	21,696	27,763
0.33	1	2	0	0	16,079	14,420	11,458	41,956*	
0.33	1	2	0	0.33	18,104	12,503	10,787	41,374	
0.33	1	2	0	0.67	18,583	10,060	9,772	38,416	
0.33	1	2	0	1	18,903	5,446	6,479	30,828	
0.33	1	2	0.33	0	18,872	8,973	6,870	34,715	
0.33	1	2	0.33	0.33	20,897	7,058	5,972	33,925	
0.33	1	2	0.33	0.67	21,377	4,614	4,661	30,651	
0.33	1	2	0.33	1	21,696	0	0	21,696	
0.33	1	0.5	0	0.33	18,104	12,503	478	31,085*	
0.33	1	0.5	0	0.6	18,583	10,060	414	29,057	
0.33	1	0.5	0	1	18,903	5,446	191	24,540	
0.33	1	0.5	0.33	0	18,872	8,973	428	28,274	
0.33	1	0.5	0.33	0.33	20,897	7,056	372	28,326	
0.33	1	0.5	0.33	0.67	21,377	4,614	291	26,281	
0.33	1	0.5	0.33	1	21,696	0	0	21,696	36,520
0.33	0.67	2	0	0	18,104	12,503	10,767	41,374*	
0.33	0.67	2	0	0.33	18,572	10,143	9,809	38,525	
0.33	0.67	2	0	0.67	18,903	5,446	6,479	30,828	
0.33	0.67	2	0.33	0	20,897	7,056	5,972	33,925	
0.33	0.67	2	0.33	0.33	21,365	4,697	4,710	30,772	
0.33	0.67	2	0.33	0.67	21,696	0	0	21,696	
0.33	0.67	0.5	0	0	18,104	12,503	478	31,085*	
0.33	0.67	0.5	0	0.33	18,572	10,143	416	29,131	
0.33	0.67	0.5	0	0.67	18,903	5,446	191	24,540	
0.33	0.67	0.5	0.33	0	20,897	7,056	372	28,326	
0.33	0.67	0.5	0.33	0.33	21,365	4,697	294	26,356	

Present Value of Benefits for Period Two Land-Use Choices ($000s)

Degree of Preservation at End of Period 1			Conversion During Period 2		Conver.	Env. Serv.	Biochem. Prosp.		Exp. Max.
Site 1	Site 2	0	Site 1	Site 2	Benefits	Benefits	Benefits	Total	Benefits
0.33	0.67	0.5	0.33	0.67	21,696	0	0	21,696	36,229
0.33	0.33	2	0	0	18,583	10,060	9,772	38,416*	
0.33	0.33	2	0	0.33	18,903	5,446	6,479	30,828	
0.33	0.33	2	0.33	0	21,377	4,614	4,661	30,651	
0.33	0.33	2	0.33	0.33	21,696	0	0	21,696	
0.33	0.33	0.5	0	0	18,583	10,060	414	29,057*	
0.33	0.33	0.5	0	0.33	18,903	5,446	191	24,540	
0.33	0.33	0.5	0.33	0	21,377	4,614	291	26,281	
0.33	0.33	0.5	0.33	0.33	21,696	0	0	21,696	33,736
0.33	0	2	0	0	18,903	446	6,479	30,828*	
0.33	0	2	0.33	0	21,696	0	0	21,696	
0.33	0	0.5	0	0	18,903	5,446	191	24,540*	
0.33	0	0.5	0.33	0	21,696	0	0	21,696	27,684
0	1	2	0	0	18,872	8,973	6,870	34,715*	
0	1	2	0	0.33	20,897	7,056	5,972	33,925	
0	1	2	0	0.67	21,377	4,614	4,661	30,651	
0	1	2	0	1	21,696	0	0	21,696	
0	1	0.5	0	0	18,872	8,973	428	28,274	
0	1	0.5	0	0.33	20,897	7,056	372	28,326*	
0	1	0.5	0	0.67	21,377	4,614	291	26,281	
0	1	0.5	0	1	21,696	0	0	21,696	31,521
0	0.67	2	0	0	20,897	7,056	5,972	33,925*	
0	0.67	2	0	0.33	21,365	4,697	4,710	30,772	
0	0.67	2	0	0.67	21,696	0	0	21,696	
0	0.67	0.5	0	0	20,897	7,056	372	28,326*	
0	0.67	0.5	0	0.33	21,365	4,697	294	26,356	
0	0.67	0.5	0	0.67	21,696	0	0	21,696	31,126
0	0.33	2	0	0	21,377	4,614	4,661	30,651*	
0	0.33	2	0	0.33	21,696	0	0	21,696	
0	0.33	0.5	0	0	21,377	4,614	291	26,281*	
0	0.33	0.5	0	0.33	21,696	0	0	21,696	28,466
0	0	2	0	0	21,696	0	0	21,696	
0	0	0.5	0	0	21,696	0	0	21,696	21,696

Notes

Chapter 1

1. They assume that half of the approximately 250,000 known species of higher plants are found in rainforest ecosystems.

2. It is interesting to contrast Simpson and colleagues' assumption that discovery of ten new drugs per year would saturate demand with Mendelsohn and Balick's estimate that each pharmaceutical company tests biological samples for 50 to 75 different therapeutic uses and the industry as a whole screens biological extracts for as many as 500 different therapeutic targets.

Chapter 2

1. In the term "biochemical prospecting organization," I include profit-seeking corporations, government research institutes, universities, and other private nonprofit organizations engaged in natural product research.

2. If the R&D process requires, for example, fourteen years to be completed, then for $t = 0$ to 14 and R_t would be zero unless a promising lead is licensed to another company.

3. The resources invested in the biochemical prospecting effort could be used for other purposes. Consequently, the social net benefits analysis must also consider whether the economic activities being foregone to pursue the prospecting effort would themselves yield benefits to society in excess of the foregone private benefits.

4. For purposes of this exposition, costs and benefits are assumed to be discounted to the start of the R&D process.

5. Biologically derived compounds that do not test positively in a particular screen or trial may still provide some benefits in the form of insights into the molecular structure of effective therapeutic agents.

6. In addition to DiMasi and colleagues, Hansen (1979) and Statman (1983) take a similar aggregate approach to estimating exploratory R&D costs.

7. In situations where a biochemical prospecting organization does not have easy access to new sources of capital, the discount rate or cost of capital should reflect the potential return available to the firm from other drug discovery opportunities, such as those posed by gene therapy or recombinatorial chemistry.

8. See Brealey and Myers (1991) for an introduction to the capital asset pricing model and its applications in corporate project analysis.

9. The market return of pharmaceutical stocks will reflect not only the expected returns on projects in various stages of R&D but also expectations about the returns on pharmaceutical products that have reached the market. It could be argued that returns on pharmaceutical R&D are more highly correlated with market returns (i.e., have a higher beta) than pharmaceutical company stock prices because ongoing R&D programs will be cut disproportionately when company revenues fall short of expectations. However, I find it more plausible to assume that research-intensive pharmaceutical companies will reduce other expenses and/or delay *new* R&D programs when faced with revenue shortfalls. This would imply that a diversified set of pharmaceutical R&D investments would have a beta value similar to that of pharmaceutical company stocks.

10. The Society for Biomolecular Screening was first organized at the Second Annual Conference on Advances in High Throughput Screening held in Princeton, NJ, April 1994.

11. Analysis of the cost estimates in the Hansen and DiMasi and colleagues studies indicate that real R&D expenditures, net of financing costs and inflation, increased by a factor of approximately 1.6 during the period 1976 to 1987. General inflationary increases from 1976 to 1987, as measured by the implicit GDP (gross domestic product) price deflator, further increased costs by a factor of 1.85. From 1987 to the end of 1994, the producer price index for pharmaceutical products increased by a factor of 1.47. To provide an updated estimate of the cost of preclinical trials, Hansen's $177,000 estimate, which was stated in 1976 dollars, has therefore been increased as follows: $177,000 × 1.6 × 1.85 × 1.47 = $771,317.

12. The DiMasi study of R&D costs is based upon a random sample of 93 new chemical entities (NCEs) first tested in humans during the period 1970–82. I have updated these cost estimates to 1995 dollars using the producer price index for drug and pharmaceutical products.

13. Grabowski and Vernon's (G&V's) study includes actual sales data through 1986, with data prior to 1986 adjusted to 1986 dollars on the basis of the GDP implicit price deflator. I have therefore adjusted G&V's sales data based on the difference between changes in the implicit GDP price deflator and the producer price index (PPI) of pharmaceutical commodities from 1975 (the midpoint of the product introduction period in the G&V study) through 1986. From 1986 through 1994, price increases are based simply on the increase in the PPI of pharmaceutical commodities.

14. These expected value estimates assume that there is no product redundancy; i.e., that the prospecting organization can substitute new therapeutic objectives if a significant number of new leads can be discovered for any one of the original ones.

15. As discussed in Chapter 4, compensation for extracts might be made as a combination of payments upon delivery and a share of the revenues or profits realized on any new drugs developed from the prospecting effort.

16. A separate decision tree would be needed to depict the value of screening each additional extract given the assumption of a declining success rate in the dereplication phase.

Chapter 3

1. Specific contractual arrangements are evaluated in Chapter 4 from both the prospecting organization's perspective and the host country's perspective.

2. The value of these other goods and services should also be included in evaluating the option of refusing the prospecting contract but preserving the proposed prospecting locations.

3. The expected benefit of preserving the site for both periods is $0.8 million + (.5 × $0.4 million) + (.5 × $1.6 million) = $1.8 million

4. This definition is an extension of the two-period analytical framework presented by Fisher and Hanemann (1986).

5. For ease of presentation, I have assumed that new information received in each time period does not affect the expected benefits of conversion of the habitat.

6. Separate random variables could be established for the value of preservation and conversion in each ecosystem, but this would greatly increase the number of possible states that must be explored in the dynamic programming analysis.

7. The quasi-option value associated with varying degrees of preservation can be computed by determining the expected value of each branch of the decision tree, assuming no change in land use can be made in Period 2, and subtracting this value from the expected value of the branch computed on the basis that feasible second-period land-use choices given P_1 are made with knowledge of $\ominus_2$.

8. The benefit functions for conversion and the environmental services of preservation implicitly assume that other inputs besides land (e.g., labor, technology) are optimized with respect to the converted or preserved land area.

9. Any additional costs for increased maintenance or protection of the prospecting location should also be deducted from the revenues of the prospecting effort.

10. If the host country has developed its own biochemical R&D program, the model developed in Chapter 2 can be used to determine the value of collecting and testing each sample.

11. INBio has embarked upon a decade-long effort to inventory all of Costa Rica's plant and animal species. In addition, Dan Janzen of the University of Pennsylvania has also been working to organize an all-species inventory of a biologically diverse site. But specimens and samples that have been or will be collected for these programs are sufficient only for taxonomic identification. Much larger samples are usually needed for biochemical screening and analysis.

12. If the number of samples to be produced is a significant fraction of current worldwide supply, it may also be necessary to estimate the market price as a function of the number of samples produced by the host country.

13. This assumption may not be entirely justified. If relatively rare species found at more than one site are relatively adaptable generalists, then partial site conversion may disproportionately affect locally unique species.

14. r_{ij} is essentially a measure of the correction between the overlapping species diversity originally found at locations i and j. If the necessary data were available, a more sophisticated analysis might use measures of phylogenetic or genetic correlation between critical species found at each site in the analysis. See, for example, Vane-Wright and colleagues (1991) and Solow and colleagues (1993).

15. Of course, if all the species that are common to more than one site are not thought to be important for purposes of biochemical prospecting or are adequately protected elsewhere, then the analysis can be simplified by focusing on only those species that are unique to each site.

16. This might be the case if the host country had entered into an exclusive contract with one prospecting organization or was screening samples as part of its own biochemical R&D program. A nonexclusive contract could be modeled using a value of v_t that reflects the market price of a sample and the expected number of prospecting organizations to which each sample could be sold.

17. For a discussion of statistical approaches that can be used to develop and revise estimates of species diversity, see Smith and van Belle (1984), Lewins and Joanes (1984), and Conroy and Smith (1994).

18. The potential benefits of regional cooperation in biochemical prospecting activities were discussed at a conference on biodiversity, biotechnology, and sustainable development sponsored by the Pan American Health Organization and the International Institute for Cooperation in Agriculture, held in Costa Rica, April 12–14, 1994, and at a conference sponsored by the International Academy of the Environment held in Cuernavaca, Mexico, April 1–4, 1994. See also Reid, Barber, and Vina (1995) for a discussion of regional approaches to biochemical prospecting.

19. This idea was first suggested to me by Dr. James McChesney of the Department of Pharmacognosy, University of Mississippi.

Chapter 4

1. This normative assumption receives some support from the absence of any exclusivity clauses in the NCI's standard Materials Transfer Agreement.

2. This equation assumes there will be no redundancy in product development, i.e., that the prospecting organization will substitute other commercial objectives if a new product or several promising leads are discovered in one or more categories.

3. If the host country is utilizing a utility function to evaluate alternative compensation arrangements, future compensation should be discounted at the riskless rate.

4. I am assuming that the prospecting organization will substitute new product objectives when a promising new lead has been discovered for any given screening target.

5. See Grabowski and Vernon (1990) for data on the distribution of new drug revenues.

6. Some data on the variability of pharmaceutical R&D costs is contained in the recent study by DiMasi and colleagues (1991).

7. This is again assuming no redundancy in product discoveries.

8. I am indebted to Paul Cox of Brigham Young University for the suggestion to explore the possible benefits of progress payments tied to successful completion of interim research phases.

9. In the unlikely case that individual product revenues are negatively correlated with success rates in each R&D phase, it is possible that the potential distribution of progress payments could have a higher variance than a royalty agreement.

10. Some correlation in returns may occur if global economic conditions affect both the price level of goods produced by the host country and the level of R&D investment of the prospecting organization.

Chapter 5

1. Biologists generally believe that there are millions of species that have not yet been discovered and named (May 1990).

2. The undertaking also sought to provide free access to the products of genetic R&D. For obvious reasons, private profit-seeking companies have been unwilling to provide free access to the fruits of their research, even if the original biological material was obtained free of charge under the rubric of common heritage (Kloppenburg and Kleinman 1988, Sedjo 1988).

3. The definition of genetic resources in the convention could be interpreted to exclude biological material that does not contain functional units of heredity. Under this interpretation, many chemical products developed from biological source material would not be governed by the convention's requirements for fair and equitable sharing of benefits.

4. Indeed, the international externalities associated with conversion of natural ecosystems are likely to be negative, even apart from the effects on biodiversity. One estimate places the costs of global warming at $13 per ton of carbon dioxide released to the atmosphere (Nordhaus 1990). Given that estimates of the carbon dioxide content of vegetation in a closed canopy forest range from 80 to 200 tons per hectare (Houghton 1990), external international costs of deforestation could be as high as $2,600 per hectare, depending on the uses to which the forest biomass are put and the vegetative cover that replaces the forest.

5. The option value of waiting to invest would be offset to some degree if a prospecting organization believed it could gain a lasting competitive advantage by being the first to establish prospecting operations within a particular country or region.

6. Ten Kate (1995, p. 35) has recommended a similar role for the clearinghouse.

7. See, for example, the declaration of Malaysia made at the adoption of the agreed text of the Convention on Biological Diversity on May 22, 1992. The Third World Network, an international NGO, has also expressed strong criticism of the intellectual property provisions of the convention and the draft U.S. interpretive statement (Shiva 1993).

8. Reid, Barber, and Vina (1995) have outlined a similar proposal for regional biological research and marketing centers. Other researchers have suggested similar compensation systems for international gene banks and agricultural research centers (Barton and Christensen 1988, pp. 348–350; Kloppenburg and Kleinman 1988).

9. Vogel (1994) has proposed that all public or private landowners that have documented the existence on their land of a species from which a new product has been generated should receive some royalty. Subramanian (1992) suggests using geographical indications or appellations of origin to allocate revenues to communal property owners.

10. To my knowledge, creation of such a fund was first proposed in a report published by the World Resources Institute (1989, p. 14).

11. Personal communication with Michael Rubino, International Finance Corporation, June 15, 1994.

12. An investment fund focused primarily on biochemical prospecting activities was proposed by Eisner and Beiring (1994). However, their original proposal emphasized the need to obtain funding for national biodiversity institutes rather than a profit-oriented investment fund.

13. By "derivative instruments" I mean contractual arrangements that provide the option, or the obligation, to buy or sell access to a particular set of biological samples of biochemical prospecting rights at a specified date or series of dates in the future.

References

Alberts, B., D. Bray, J. Lewis, M. Raff, K. Roberts, and J.D. Watson. 1989. *The Molecular Biology of the Cell*, Second Edition. New York: Garland Publishing.

Anderson, J.E., C.M. Goetz, J.L. McLaughlin, and M. Suffness. 1991. A Blind Comparison of Simple Bench—Top Bioassays and Human Tumor Cell Cytotoxicities as Antitumor Prescreens. *Phytochemical Analysis*. 90:107–111.

Armond, P.A. 1994. Beyond the Romance of Plants: Deciding to Invest in Medicinal Plant Programs. Presentation to the Conference on Drug Discovery and Commercial Opportunities in Medicinal Plants. September 19–20, 1994. Washington, DC.

Arrow, K.J. 1963. *Social Choice and Individual Values*. New York: Wiley.

Arrow, K.J. 1984. *The Economics of Information. Vol. 4. The Collected Papers of Kenneth J. Arrow*. Cambridge, MA: Belknap Press.

Arrow, K.J., and A.C. Fisher. 1974. Environmental Preservation, Uncertainty and Irreversibility. *Quarterly Journal of Economics*. 88:312–319.

Arrow, K.J., and R.C. Lind. 1970. Uncertainty and the Evaluation of Public Investment Decisions. *American Economic Review*. 60:364–378.

Asebey, E.J. 1996. Andes Pharmaceuticals, Inc.: A New Model for Biodiversity Prospecting. In J. Feinsilver (ed.) *Emerging Connections: Biodiversity, Biotechnology, and Sustainable Development in Health and Agriculture*. Washington, DC: Pan American Health Organization.

Aylward, B.A. 1993. *The Economic Value of Pharmaceutical Prospecting and Its Role in Biodiversity Conservation*. LEEC Paper DP 93–103. London: London Environmental Economics Centre.

Aylward, B.A., and E.B. Barbier. 1992. *What Is Biodiversity Worth to a Developing Country?* LEEC Paper DP 92–105. London: London Environmental Economics Centre.

Balick, M.J. 1990. Ethnobotany and the Identification of Therapeutic Agents from the Rainforest. In *Bioactive Compounds from Plants*. (Ciba Foundation Symposium 154). Chichester, UK: Wiley, pp. 22–39.

Balthasar, H.U., R.A.A. Boschi, and M.M. Menke. 1978. Calling the Shots in R&D. *Harvard Business Review*. May–June:151–160.

Barton, J.H., and E. Christensen. 1988. Diversity Compensation Systems: Ways to Compensate Developing Nations for Providing Genetic Material. In *Seeds and Sovereignty*. J.R. Kloppenburg, Jr., (ed.). Durham, NC: Duke University Press, pp. 339–355.

Barzel, Y. 1982. Measurement Costs and the Organization of Markets. *Journal of Law and Economics*. 25:27–48.

Bent, S.A., R.L. Schwaab, D.G. Conlin, and D.D. Jeffery. 1987. *Intellectual Property Rights in Biotechnology Worldwide.* New York: Stockton Press.

Bibby, C.J., N.J. Collar, and M.J. Crosby. 1992. *Putting Biodiversity on the Map: Priority Areas for Global Conservation.* Cambridge: International Council for Bird Preservation.

Borris, R.P. 1994. Industrial Pharmacognosy in the 1990's. Presentation to the Conference on Drug Discovery and Commercial Opportunities in Medicinal Plants. September 19 – 20, 1994. Washington, DC.

Brealy, R., and S. Myers. 1991. *Principles of Corporate Finance.* New York: McGraw Hill.

Broad, W.J. 1993. Strange Oases in Sea Depths Offer Map to Riches. *New York Times.* November 16, C1.

Brown, K.S., and G.G. Brown. 1992. Habitat Alteration and Species Loss in Brazilian Forests. In: *Tropical Deforestation and Species Extinction.* T.C. Whitmore and J.A. Sayer, eds. London: Chapman and Hall, pp. 119 – 142.

Burger, A. 1990. Drug Design. In: *Drug Development.* C.E. Hamner (ed.). Boca Raton, FL: CRC Press, pp. 39 – 50.

Caporale, L. 1994. Drug Discovery and Biodiversity: Collaborations and Risk in the Discovery of New Pharmaceuticals. Paper presented at the Conference on Biodiversity, Biotechnology, and Sustainable Development. Organized by Pan American Health Organization and International Institute for Cooperation in Agriculture. April 13 – 15, 1994. San Jose, Costa Rica

Chien, R.I., and R.B. Upson. 1980. Returns to Drug Industry Common Stock. *Managerial and Decision Economics.* 1:172 – 178.

Clemente, C. 1988. A Pharmaceutical Industry Perspective. In *Intellectual Property Rights and Capital Formation in the Next Decade.* C. Walker and M. Bloomfield, eds. Lanham, MD: University Press of America.

Connor, E.F., and E.D. McCoy. 1979. The Statistics and Biology of the Species-Area Relationship. *American Naturalist.* 113:791 – 833.

Conroy, M.J., and D.R. Smith. 1994. Designing Large Scale Surveys of Wildlife Abundance and Diversity Using Statistical Sampling Principles. *Trans. North American Wildlife Natural Resource Conference.* 59:159 – 169.

Correa, C.M. 1991. The Pharmaceutical Industry and Biotechnology: Opportunities and Constraints for Developing Countries. *World Competition.* 15(2):43 – 63.

Cox, C.J., and M. Rubenstein. 1985. *Options Markets.* Englewood Cliffs, NJ: Prentice Hall.

Devlin, J.P. 1995. Compound Libraries as a Discovery Resource. *Screening Forum.* 3(1):11.

DiMasi, J.A., R.W. Hansen, H.G. Grabowski, and L. Lasagna. 1991. Cost of Innovation in the Pharmaceutical Industry. *Journal of Health Economics.* 10:107 – 142.

Eisner, T., and E.A. Beiring. 1994. Biotic Exploration Fund: Protecting Biodiversity Through Chemical Prospecting. *Bioscience.* 44:95 – 98.

FAO. 1990. *Interim Report on Forest Resources Assessment.* Rome: FAO Committee on Forestry, 10th Session. COFO – 90/8(a).

Farnsworth, N.R., and D.D. Soejarto. 1985. Potential Consequences of Plant Extinction in the U. S. on the Availability of Prescription Drugs. *Economic Botany.* 39(3):231–240.

Fisher, A., and W.M. Hanemann. 1986. Option Value and the Extinction of Species. In *Advances in Applied Microeconomics.* Vol. 4. Greenwich, CT: JAI Press.

Fisher, A., and W.M. Hanemann. 1987. Quasi-Option Value: Some Misconceptions Dispelled. *Journal of Environmental Economics and Management.* 14:183–190.

Food and Drug Administration (FDA). 1988. *From Test Tube to Patient: New Drug Development in the United States.* Washington, DC: FDA.

Freeman, A.M. 1984. The Quasi-Option Value of Irreversible Development. *Journal of Environmental Management.* 11:292–295.

French, K.R., and R.E. McCormick. 1984. Sealed Bids, Sunk Costs, and the Process of Competition. *Journal of Business.* 57:417–441.

Gericke, N. 1994. Traditional Medicines Program. South Africa: University of Cape Town.

Grabowski, H., and J. Vernon. 1990. A New Look at the Returns and Risks to Pharmaceutical R&D. *Management Science.* 36:804–821.

Grifo, F. 1996. Chemical Prospecting: An Overview of the International Cooperative Biodiversity Groups Program. In *Emerging Connections: Biodiversity, Biotechnology, and Sustainable Development.* J. Feinsilver, ed. Pan American Health Organization. Washington, DC.

Grifo, F.T., D. Newman, A. Fairfield, J.T. Grupenhoff, and B. Bhattacharya. 1996. The Origins of Prescription Drugs. In *Biodiversity and Human Health.* F.T. Griffo and J. Rosenthal, eds. Washington, DC: Island Press.

Haagsma, A. 1988. A View from the European Community. In *Intellectual Property Rights and Capital Formation in the Next Decade.* C. Walker and M. Bloomfield, eds. Lanham, MD: University Press of America.

Hammond, P. 1992. Species Inventory. In *Global Biodiversity.* B. Groombridge (ed.). London: World Conservation Monitoring Centre and Chapman & Hall, pp. 17–39.

Hansen, R.W. 1979. The Pharmaceutical Development Process: Estimates of Development Costs and Times. In *Issues in Pharmaceutical Health Economics.* R.I. Chien, ed. Lexington, MA: Lexington Books.

Harcourt, C. 1992. Tropical Moist Forests. In: *Global Biodiversity.* B. Groombridge, ed. London: World Conservation Monitoring Centre and Chapman & Hall, pp. 256–275.

Harris, A. 1995. Improving Molecular Diversity of a Compound Collection in a High Throughput Screening Program. *The Society for Biomolecular Screening Newsline.* 1:3.

Hausman, J.A. 1993. *Contingent Valuation: A Critical Assessment.* Amsterdam: North Holland.

Hawksworth, D.L. 1992. Microorganisms. In *Global Biodiversity.* B. Groombridge, ed. London: World Conservation Monitoring Centre and Chapman & Hall, pp. 47–54.

Henry, C. 1974. Investment Decisions Under Uncertainty: The Irreversibility Effect. *American Economic Review.* 64:1007 – 1112.

Heywood, V.H., and S.N. Stuart. 1992. Species Extinctions in Tropical Forests. In *Tropical Deforestation and Species Extinction.* T.C. Whitmore and J.A. Sayer (eds.). London: Chapman and Hall, pp. 91 – 118.

Houghten, R.A. 1988. Methods for Rapid Synthesis of Large Numbers of Discrete Peptides. In *Macromolecular Sequencing and Synthesis: Selected Methods and Applications.* D. H. Schlesinger, ed. New York: Alan R. Liss, pp. 185 – 194.

Houghton, R.A. 1990. The Future Role of Tropical Forests in Affecting Carbon Dioxide Concentration of the Atmosphere. *Ambio.* 19:204 – 209.

Hunter, M.L., Jr. 1991. Coping with Ignorance: The Coarse Filter Strategy for Maintaining Biodiversity. In *Balancing on the Brink of Extinction.* K.A. Kohm (ed.). Washington, DC: Island Press, pp. 266 – 281.

Ibbotson, R.G., and R.A. Sinquefeld. 1988. *Stocks, Bonds, Bills, and Inflation 1926 – 1987.* Charlottesville, VA: Research Foundation of Institute of Chartered Financial Analysts.

Instituto Nacional de Biodiversidad (INBio). 1992a. Una Lucha Contra la Malaria. *Informa.* July 1992. Heredia, Costa Rica: INBio.

INBio. 1992b. Excelentes Resultados Arrojan Plantas Nematicidas. *Informa.* July 1992. Heredia, Costa Rica: INBio.

INBio. 1992c. Una Esperanza para Combatir Trombosis. *Informa.* July 1992. Heredia, Costa Rica: INBio.

Janzen, D.H. 1986. The Eternal External Threat. In *Conservation Biology: The Science of Scarcity and Diversity.* M.E. Soule, ed. Sunderland, MA: Sinauer Assoc., pp. 286 – 313.

Janzen, D.H. 1991. How to Save Tropical Biodiversity. *American Entomologist.* 37(Fall):159 – 71.

Janzen, D.H., W. Hallwachs, R. Gamez, A. Sittenfeld, and J. Jiminez. 1993. Research Management Policies: Permits for Research and Collecting in the Tropics. In *Biodiversity Prospecting.* W.V. Reid et al. (eds.). Washington, DC: World Resources Institute, pp. 131 – 158.

Jensen, E.J. 1987. Research Expenditures and the Discovery of New Drugs. *Journal of Industrial Economics.* 36:83 – 95.

Joglekar, P., and M.L. Paterson. 1986. A Closer Look at the Returns and Risks of Pharmaceutical R&D. *Journal of Health Economics.* 5:153 – 77.

Johns, A.D. 1992. Species Conservation in Managed Tropical Forests. In *Tropical Deforestation and Species Extinction.* T.C. Whitmore and J.A. Sayer (eds.). London: Chapman and Hall, pp. 15 – 54.

Johns, R.J. 1992. The Influence of Deforestation and Selective Logging Operations on Plant Diversity in New Guinea. In *Tropical Deforestation and Species Extinction.* T.C. Whitmore and J.A. Sayer (eds.). London: Chapman and Hall, pp. 15–54.

Joyce, G.F. 1992. Directed Molecular Evolution. *Scientific American.* 267(6):90 – 97.

Juma, C. 1993. Policy Options for Scientific and Technological Capacity—Building. In *Biodiversity Prospecting*. W.V. Reid et al. (eds.). Washington, DC: World Resources Institute.

King, S.R., and M.S. Tempesta. 1993. *From Shaman to Human Clinical Trials*. Ciba Foundation Symposium No. 185. Amsterdam: Associated Scientific Publishers.

Klocke, J.A. 1989. Plant Compounds as a Source and Models of Insect-Control Agents. In *Economic and Medicinal Plant Research*. H. Wagner, H. Hikino, and N. Farnsworth (eds.). 3:104 – 144. London: Academic Press Limited.

Kloppenburg, J.R., Jr., and D.L. Kleinman. 1988. Seeds of Controversy: National Property vs. Common Heritage. In *Seeds and Sovereignty*. J.R. Kloppenburg (ed.). Durham, NC: Duke University Press, pp. 173 – 203.

Kloppenburg, J.R., Jr. 1988. *First the Seed: The Political Economy of Plant Biotechnology, 1492 – 2000*. Cambridge: Cambridge University Press.

Kricher, J.C. 1989. *A Neotropical Companion*. Princeton: Princeton University Press.

Laird, S.A. 1993. Contracts for Biodiversity Prospecting. In *Biodiversity Prospecting*. W.V. Reid et al. (eds.). Washington, DC: World Resources Institute, pp. 99 – 131.

Leary, W.E. 1993. Science Takes a Lesson from Nature: Imitating Abalone and Spider Silk. *New York Times*. August 31, C1.

Leffler, K.B., and R.R. Rucker. 1991. Transaction Costs and the Efficient Organization of Production: A Study of Timber-Harvesting Contracts. *Journal of Political Economy*. 99:1060 – 1087.

Lesser, W.H., and A.F. Krattiger. 1994. Marketing "Genetic Technologies" in South-North and South-South Exchanges: The Proposed Role of a New Facilitating Organisation. In *Widening Perspectives on Biodiversity*. Geneva, Switzerland: IUCN. Gland Switzerland & International Academy for the Environment.

Lewins, W.A., and D.N. Joanes. 1984. Bayesian Estimation of the Number of Species. *Biometrics*. 40:323 – 328.

Lipton, R.J. 1995. DNA Solution of Hard Computational Problems. *Science*. 268(5210):542 – 545.

Loll, P.J., D. Picot, and R.M. Garavito. 1995. The structural basis of aspirin activity inferred from crystal structure of inactivated prostaglandin H_2 synthase. *Nature Structural Biology*. 2(8):637 – 643.

Lovejoy, T.E. 1980. A Projection of Species Extinctions. In *Global 2000 Report to the President*. 2:328 – 331. Washington, DC: Council on Environmental Quality.

Lovejoy, T.E., R.O. Bierregaard, A.B. Rylands, J.R. Malcolm, C.E. Quintela, L.H. Harper, K.S. Brown, A.H. Powell, G.V.N. Powell, H.O.R. Schubart, and M.B. Hays. 1986. Edge and Other Effects of Isolation on Amazon Forest Fragments. In *Conservation Biology: The Science of Scarcity and Diversity*. M.E. Soule (ed.). Sunderland, MA: Sinauer Assoc., pp. 257 – 285.

Luce, D.R., and H. Raiffa. 1957. *Games and Decisions*. New York: Wiley & Sons.

Mansfield, E. 1992. Unauthorized Use of Intellectual Property: Effects on Investment, Technology Transfer and Innovation. In *Global Dimensions of Intellectual Property Rights in Science and Technology*. M.B. Wallerstein, M.E. Mogee, and R.A. Schoen (eds.). Washington, DC: National Research Council, National Academy Press, pp. 107 – 145.

Mansfield, E., J. Rappaport, A. Romeo, S. Wagner, and G. Beardsley. 1977. Social and Private Rates of Return from Industrial Innovations. *Quarterly Journal of Economics*. May: 221 – 240.

Margules, C.R, A.O. Nicoll, and R.L. Pressey. 1988. Selecting Networks of Reserves to Maximize Conservation. *Biological Conservation*. 43:63 – 76.

May, R.M. 1990. How Many Species? *Philosophical Transactions of the Royal Society*. B330:293 – 304.

McNeil, R.J., and M.J. McNeil. 1989. Ownership of Traditional Information. *Northeast Indian Quarterly*. Fall. 30 – 35.

Mendelsohn, R., and M.J. Balick. 1995. The Value of Undiscovered Pharmaceuticals in Tropical Forests. *Economic Botany*. 49(2):223 – 228.

Mitscher, L.A., S. Drake, S.R. Gollapudi, and S.K. Okwute. 1987. A Modern Look at Folkloric Use of Anti-Infective Agents. *Journal of Natural Products*. 50(6): 1025 – 1040.

Moran, K. 1995. Returning Benefits from Drug Discoveries to Local Communities. Paper presented at the Biodiversity and Human Health Conference. Smithsonian Institute. April 3 – 5, 1995. Washington, DC.

Myers, N. 1988. Threatened Biotas: Hot Spots in Tropical Forests. *The Environmentalist*. 8(3):187 – 208.

Myers, N. 1990. The Biodiversity Challenge: Expanded Hot Spots Analysis. *The Environmentalist*. 10(4):243 – 255.

Myers, N. 1992. *The Primary Source*. New York: Norton & Co.

National Cancer Institute (NCI). 1994. *Cancer Facts: Questions and Answers About NCI's Natural Products Branch*. Washington, DC: National Institutes of Health.

National Research Council (NRC). 1992. *Conserving Biodiversity: A Research Agenda for Development Agencies*. Washington, DC: National Academy Press.

Nordhaus, W. 1990. To Slow or Not to Slow: The Economics of the Greenhouse Effect. Working paper. New Haven, CT: Department of Economics, Yale University.

Oldfield, M.L. 1984. *The Value of Conserving Genetic Resources*. Washington, DC: U.S. Department of the Interior, National Park Service.

Pharmaceutical Manufacturers Association (PMA). 1985. *Modern Medicines: Saving Lives and Money*. Washington, DC: PMA.

PMA. 1992. *Cost Effectiveness of Pharmaceuticals*. Industry Issue Brief. July. Washington, DC: PMA.

Pindyck, R.S. 1991. Irreversibility, Uncertainty and Investment. *Journal of Economic Literature*. 29:1110 – 1148.

Pollock, A. 1992. Drug Industry Going Back to Nature. *New York Times*. March 3, D1.

Principe, P.P. 1989. The Economic Significance of Plants and Their Constituents as Drugs. In *Economic and Medicinal Plant Research*. Vol. 3. H. Wagner, H. Hikino, and N.R. Farnsworth, eds. San Diego: Academic Press.

Ramsey, J.R. 1980. *Bidding and Oil Leases*. Contemporary Studies in Economic and Financial Analysis. Vol. 25. Greenwich, CT: JAI Press.

Raven, P.H. 1988. Our Diminishing Tropical Forests. In *Biodiversity*. E.O. Wilson, ed. Washington, DC: National Academy Press, pp. 119 – 122.

Raven, P.H., and E.O. Wilson. 1992. A Fifty Year Plan for Biodiversity Surveys. *Science*. 258:1099 – 1100.

Reid, W.V. 1992. How Many Species Will There Be? In *Tropical Deforestation and Species Extinction*. T.C. Whitmore and J.A. Sayer (eds.). London: Chapman and Hall, pp. 55 – 74.

Reid, W.V., S.A. Laird, R. Gamez, A. Sittenfeld, D.H. Janzen, M.A. Gollin, and C. Juma. 1993. A New Lease on Life. In *Biodiversity Prospecting*. W.V. Reid et al. (eds.). Washington, DC: World Resources Institute, pp. 1 – 52.

Reid, W.V., C.V. Barber, and A.L. Vina. 1995. Translating Genetic Resource Rights into Sustainable Development: Gene Cooperatives, the Biotrade and Lessons from the Philippines. *Plant Genetic Resources Newsletter*. (102):1 – 17.

Rosenthal, J. 1995. *Progress Report on International Cooperative Biodiversity Group Program*. Washington, DC: Fogarty International Center, National Institutes of Health.

Royal Botanic Gardens, Kew. 1994. *Plantas do Nordeste: Local Plants for Local People*. Kew, UK.

Rubeck, J.R., Jr. 1994. Synthetic Self-Replicating Molecules. *Scientific American*. 271(1):48 – 55.

Saunders, D.A., R.J. Hobbs, and C.R. Margules. 1991. Biological Consequences of Ecosystem Fragmentation: A Review. *Conservation Biology*. 5:18 – 32.

Schelhas, J. 1994. *Forest Patches in the Tropical Landscape*. Washington, DC: Smithsonian Migratory Bird Center.

Scott, J.M., B. Csuti, K. Smith, J.E. Estes, and S. Caico. 1991. Gap Analysis of Species Richness and Vegetation Cover. In *Balancing on the Brink of Extinction*. K.A. Kohm (ed.). Washington, DC: Island Press.

Sebenius, J.K., and P.J.E. Stan. 1982. Risk-Spreading Properties of Common Tax and Contract Instruments. *Bell Journal of Economics*. 13:555 – 560.

Sedjo, R.A. 1988. Property Rights and the Protection of Plant Genetic Resources. In *Seeds and Sovereignty*. J.R. Kloppenburg (ed.). Durham, NC: Duke University Press, pp. 293 – 314.

Sherwood, R.M. 1990. *Intellectual Property and Economic Development*. Boulder, CO: Westview Press.

Sherwood, R.M. 1992. Why Uniform Intellectual Property System Makes Sense for the World. In *Global Dimensions of Intellectual Property Rights in Science and Technology*. M.B. Wallerstein, M.E. Mogee, and R.A. Schoen (eds.). Washington, DC: National Research Council and National Academy Press, pp. 68 – 88.

Shiva, V. 1993. Intellectual Property Rights May Block Biodiversity Conservation. Third World Network Briefing Paper. Text of speech delivered at International Seminar on Biodiversity Convention. Trondheim, Norway. New Delhi: Third World Network.

Simberloff, D. 1986. Are We on the Verge of a Mass Extinction in Tropical Rain Forests. In *Dynamics of Extinction*. D.K. Elliot (ed.). New York: Wiley, pp. 165 – 180.

Simberloff, D. 1992. Do Species-Area Curves Predict Extinction in Fragmented Forests? In *Tropical Deforestation and Species Extinction*. T.C. Whitmore and J.A. Sayer (eds.). London: Chapman and Hall, pp. 75 – 89.

Simpson, R.D., R.A. Sedjo, J.W. Reid. 1996. Valuing Biodiversity for Use in Pharmaceutical Research. *Journal of Political Economy*. 104:1548 –1570.

Sittenfeld, A., and R. Gamez. 1993. Biodiversity Prospecting by INBio. In *Biodiversity Prospecting*. W.V. Reid et al. (eds.). Washington, DC: World Resources Institute, pp. 69 – 97.

Smith, E.P., and G. van Belle. 1984. Nonparametric Estimation of Species Richness. *Biometrics*. 40:119 – 129.

Smith, J.E., and R.F. Nau. 1992. Valuing Risky Projects: Option Pricing Theory and Decision Analysis. Working Paper #9201. Durham, NC: Fuqua School of Business, Duke University.

Soejarto, D., and N. Farnsworth. 1989. Tropical Rainforests: Potential Sources of New Drugs. *Perspectives in Biology and Medicine*. 33:244 – 256.

Solow, A., S. Polasky, and J. Broadus. 1993. On the Measurement of Biological Diversity. *Journal of Environmental Economics and Management*. 24:60 – 68.

Soule, M.E., and K.A. Kohm. 1989. *Research Priorities for Conservation Biology*. Washington, DC: Island Press.

Statman, M. 1983. *Competition in the Pharmaceutical Industry*. Washington, DC: American Enterprise Institute.

Stork, N.E. 1988. Insect Diversity: Facts, Fiction and Speculation. *Biological Journal of the Linnean Society*. 35:321 – 337.

Subramanian, A. 1992. Genetic Resources. Biodiversity and Environmental Protection. *Journal of World Trade*. 26:105 – 109.

Suffness, M., and J. Douros. 1982. Current Status of the NCI Plant and Animal Product Program. *Journal of Natural Products*. 45:1 – 14.

Ten Kate, K. 1995. *BioPiracy or Green Petroleum?* Report prepared for the Overseas Development Administration. London.

Thompson, J. 1996. Marine Bioprospecting. In *Biodiversity and Human Health*. Washington, DC: Island Press.

Tyler, V.E., R. Lynn, and J.E. Robbers. 1988. *Pharmacognosy*, Ninth Edition. Philadelphia: Lea & Febiger.

United Nations Centre on Transnational Corporations. 1983. *Main Features and Trends in Petroleum and Mining Agreements*. New York: United Nations.

United Nations Conference on Trade and Development (UNCTAD). 1995. Statement to the Second Conference of the Parties Convention on Biological Diversity, Jakarta. November 15, 1995.

United Nations Environment Program (UNEP). June 1992. *Convention on Biological Diversity*. Na.92 – 8314. Nairobi: UNEP, Environmental Law and Institutions Programme.

U.S. International Trade Commission (USITC). 1991. Global Competitiveness of U.S. Advanced Technology Manufacturing Industries: Pharmaceuticals. *World Competition*. 15(2):27 – 45.

Vagelos, P.R. 1991. Are Prescription Drug Prices Too High? *Science*. 252:1080 – 1084.

Vane-Wright, R.I., P.H. Humphries, and P.H. Williams. 1991. What to Protect?—Systematics and the Agony of Choice. *Biological Conservation*. 55: 235 – 254.

Vogel, J.H. 1994. *Genes for Sale: Privatisation as a Conservation Policy.* New York: Oxford University Press.

Weisbrod, B.A. 1964. Collective Consumption Services of Individual Consumption Goods. *Quarterly Journal of Economics.* 78:471 – 477.

Whitmore, T.C., and J.A. Sayer. 1992. Deforestation and Species Extinction in Tropical Moist Forests. In *Tropical Deforestation and Species Extinction.* T.C. Whitmore and J.A. Sayer, eds. London: Chapman and Hall, pp. 1 – 14.

World Conservation Monitoring Centre (WCMC). 1992. *Global Biodiversity: Status of the Earth's Living Resources.* London: Chapman & Hall.

World Resources Institute (WRI). 1989. *Natural Endowments: Financing Resource Conservation for Development.* Washington, DC: World Resources Institute.

Wu, S.Y. 1984. Social and Private Returns Derived from Pharmaceutical Innovations: Some Empirical Findings. In *Arne Ryde Symposium on Pharmaceutical Economics.* Bjorn Lindgren (ed.). Swedish Institute for Health Economics and Liber Forlag.

Index

Pages numbers followed by the letter "i" indicate illustrations; those followed by the letter "t" indicate tables.